The CAN-DO EATING PLAN
for OVERWEIGHT KIDS and TEENS

The CAN-DO EATING PLAN for OVERWEIGHT KIDS and TEENS

Helping Kids Control Weight, Look Better, and Feel Great

Michelle Daum, M.S., R.D.
with Amy Lemley

AVON BOOKS ◆ NEW YORK

AVON BOOKS
A division of
The Hearst Corporation
1350 Avenue of the Americas
New York, New York 10019

Library of Congress Cataloging in Publication Data:
Daum, Michelle.
    The Can-Do Eating Plan for Overweight Kids and Teens / Michelle Daum.
        p.   cm.
1. Obesity in children—Prevention.   2. Overweight children—
Nutrition.   3. Children—Nutrition.   4. Consumer education.   I. Title.
RJ399.C6D38   1997   96-25742
613.2'5'083—dc20   CIP

First Avon Books Trade Printing: March 1997

AVON TRADEMARK REG. U.S. PAT. OFF. AND IN OTHER COUNTRIES, MARCA REGISTRADA,
HECHO EN U.S.A.

Printed in the U.S.A.

OPM   10 9 8 7 6 5 4 3 2 1

All children are unique, and this book is not intended to substitute for the advice of your pediatrician or other health care professional, especially when a child shows any sign of illness or unusual behavior. In fact, consulting with your child's physician is an essential first step in determining the extent of your child's excess weight problem and in selecting an appropriate level of calorie intake.

Contents

Introduction

In fifteen years as a pediatric nutritionist, I have worked with hundreds of overweight children and their parents. They come to me in search of answers. "*Is* my child overweight?" "Will he grow out of it?" "What can we do?" Weight struggles are a difficult challenge for anyone, especially children. I developed the *Can-Do Eating Plan for Overweight Kids and Teens* so that children in need of weight management can eat sensibly and burn those extra calories while still enjoying the foods they love. On my program, your child can say yes to treats such as candy and cookies, go to pizza parties and celebrate birthdays with the rest of the kids—and still get his weight problem under control. This clinically proven, nutritionally balanced plan allows your child to enjoy the foods of childhood while maintaining the proper calorie intake for his or her needs.

Many parents come to me frustrated, having "tried everything" to control their child's weight. "I buy fruits and vegetables, but my daughter won't touch them," they say. Or "I've talked with my son about giving up sweets, but I'm still finding candy wrappers around the house."

I understand. I'm a parent, too, and I've faced similar frustrations. My own experience as a parent first began when I married my husband, who had an eight-year-old daughter and a twelve-year-old son. My dreams of health-food-loving, junk-food-hating children were quickly shattered, for here were real live children with ideas of their own. Michael would eat only one green vegetable: string beans. And Sara kept a stash of candy to rival any trick-or-treater's. Sure, over time the kids changed a little, but I changed, too; I learned how to nourish them well and still let them be kids. Fruits and veggies are great, but there has to be room for chips and ice cream, too. In time, our family grew to include five children, my two step-children and the three children we have had together, ranging in age from two to twenty-four. And I've gotten to know hundreds of other kids through my practice.

Children's nutrition has been the focus of my career from the start. After receiving a master's degree in nutrition from Columbia University, I completed a fellowship in pediatric nutrition at Johns Hopkins University Medical Center. Later, as the chief clinical nutritionist for the Pediatric Obesity Center at North Shore University Hospital–Cornell University Medical College, I began to realize that traditional weight-control diets simply do not work for children. The foods diets allow are not the foods kids want to eat. Applying the lessons I had learned as a parent, I gradually developed a different kind of weight-control program, one that is nutritionally balanced *and* kid-pleasing because it includes an appetizing, varied list of choices throughout the day—with many childhood favorites as part of the daily menus; and plenty of snacks—the good stuff, not just carrots and celery.

From the moment my patients hear about my menus and product guide, they express two feelings—relief that I will not be taking away all the foods they like to eat and excitement that this plan really will work. And it does. Time and time again, I have seen kids' lives transformed as they bring their weight under control, gain self-confidence, and enjoy childhood.

Why Wait?

Many parents have told me that it doesn't feel right not to feed a child who says she's hungry. If your child asks for food, how do you say no? Parents fear that their children will be hungry, miserable, and angry if they try to limit food intake. What parents don't always realize is that children ask for food for many different reasons besides hunger, including frustration, loneliness and even boredom. Don't worry. With this balanced plan, which includes three meals a day and snacks, your child will get plenty to eat.

Of course, setting limits is hard for parents to do under any circumstances. And when it comes to meeting a child's basic need for food, parents tend to worry. What if Jamie's still hungry? Did Matthew get enough protein? Shouldn't Emily have another piece of fruit today? Parents are afraid that limiting what their children eat will cause physical harm. They may also fear drawing attention to the unpleasant topic of being overweight. There are many reasons some parents resist putting their child on any sort of eating plan. But the Can-Do Eating Plan is risk-free. In using this program, you will learn how much food is enough and where to draw the line. And you don't have to be a nutritionist to understand it.

Whatever the reason, some parents wait a lot longer than they need to before seeking help for their child's weight problem. Parents often tell me their family doctor or pediatrician never raised the issue, leading them to believe there is nothing to worry about, or that they should leave their child alone. But improving your child's self-esteem by helping him to control his weight will promote emotional and physical health. The time to act is now, before your child spends another day feeling that overweight is just the way things are for him.

Who Is This Program For?

This program is designed for children ages five through eighteen, boys and girls alike. Teens are ready to take charge of their own weight management, and chapter 9 was written especially for them. It's important to realize that not every overweight child needs to lose weight, nor must those who need to lose weight do so in a hurry. Some children may simply need to slow down their weight gain, or remain at the same weight while growing. In a single medical visit, you and your child's health professional can determine where your child fits in and set reasonable goals to help her achieve and maintain an appropriate weight.

Why I Wrote *The Can-Do Eating Plan for Overweight Kids and Teens*

In general, a nutrition consultation with an overweight child takes an enormous amount of time and input—time doctors may not be able to offer and parents may not be able to afford. And really, that is why I wrote this book: To give parents and children a place to turn for a good, practical eating strategy they can implement themselves, without the fighting, without the heartache, without the bother of conventional diets.

Seeing an unhappy, underconfident overweight child blossom into a happy, healthy individual with improved self-esteem is an extraordinary experience. In learning to manage a weight problem, a child not only gains emotional and physical health benefits, but also learns that he or she can set a goal and attain it. Parents benefit too: Gone are the daily struggles about food. Gone are the feelings of guilt or shame over "not doing enough" to help an overweight child. The program I have developed takes the conflict and deprivation out of weight management, replacing it with a truly liveable, workable plan that kids really like. The Can-Do Eating Plan is a program for life. It can see you and your child through year after year of birthdays, holidays, vacations, and all the occasions worth celebrating.

I am so glad to have written *The Can-Do Eating Plan for Overweight Kids and Teens.* This information has already helped hundreds of children, and I hope that this book will help many more. This revolutionary program is easy to follow and really works. "My" kids like it and I believe yours will, too.

The CAN-DO EATING PLAN for OVERWEIGHT KIDS and TEENS

1

The Weight Is Over:
How This Book Can Help Your Overweight Child

*"I've been concerned about Mark's weight for a while.
But I'm afraid to mention it to him. I was always called
'fat' when I was growing up, and it's still hard to think
about it. I don't want to hurt his feelings."*

*"I know I probably should make sure Jenny eats a
little less. But she usually makes a scene when she
doesn't get her way, and I'm afraid of adding to the
family tension."*

*"I don't want to limit Andrea's food at mealtimes.
What if she doesn't get enough of what she needs to
grow?"*

Until now, you may have hesitated to do anything about your
child's weight problem. Like Mark's, Jenny's, and Andrea's
parents, you've been worried about your child. You want to do
the right thing. You're just not sure what that is.

You're not alone.

Many of the parents who consult with me are concerned
about the risks—not the risks of their child being overweight,
but the risks of putting their child on a "diet." You may feel
the same way they do. Like them, you may be:

- unsure whether your child really wants help
- afraid you'll have to deprive or "starve" your child to get
  results

- worried that drawing attention to the problem will make your child feel bad
- uncomfortable saying no to requests for food
- hopeful—yet doubtful—that your child will grow out of it
- confused and overwhelmed at the prospect of making the right choices in the supermarket
- at your wit's end—because you just don't know how to help

Let me end your worries right now:

I devised the *Can-Do Eating Plan* to show you the way to balance sensible, good-for-you foods with a variety of treats in a way that is easy to follow, now and for a lifetime.

Because it's designed specifically for kids, my program focuses on the fun of childhood and not the drudgery of dieting. You will love it. Your child will love it. And it will work. If you follow the guidelines in this book, your worries about your overweight child are over. Here's why:

1. Your overweight child absolutely wants help. In fifteen years of practice, I have never met an overweight child who didn't want to try this plan. Once I explain how it works, they are usually eager to get started. Why? Because they are unhappy being overweight. That's the bottom line.

Each overweight child is different, but they all have some things in common. The kids I've worked with:

- hate "being fat"
- are embarrassed about how they look
- feel alone with this problem
- think their friends can eat whatever they want without gaining weight
- feel their weight interferes in their life, affecting their friendships and preventing them from doing things they'd like to do

- have been teased or ridiculed by other kids
- feel sad about the way they are treated by other kids
- have been struggling with the problem for a while
- are frustrated by their unsuccessful efforts at weight management
- jump at the chance to correct the problem

To a ten-year-old, the health risks of adult obesity are an eternity away. But the desire to socialize—to make friends, have fun, to feel accepted and valued—is ever-present. When I talk with my patients about their peer relationships, they often dissolve into tears as they remember their "hurts." Children want to be part of the group. When something prevents that, the pain is devastating.

Most overweight children are bothered by their weight, even if they deny that they are troubled by it, even if they don't talk about it, even if they don't ask for help. Give them the opportunity—in the form of a simple, easy-to-follow program that really will work—and they will do all they can to help solve their weight problem.

When should you address your child's overweight? Look to your child's doctor, school nurse, teacher, and even yourself for the answer. But also, and most important, pay attention to your child. *Listen.* If he says he feels slow, clumsy, tired, if he won't play the sports his friends are playing, if he complains of schoolmates teasing him about his weight—then the time has come. He wants and needs your help.

2. You will not have to "starve" your child to get results. Parents often hesitate to address a child's weight problem for fear of depriving their child of essential nutrients. But my plan limits your child's calorie intake without jeopardizing his nutritional balance. It is normal for children to get their daily caloric requirements by eating three meals a day and a few snacks. On this plan, there is no need to limit between-meal snacking or restrict your child to "health foods" only. There is room for both the good-for-you foods and the snack foods kids love. This plan takes your child's eating habits into account in a way that lets life go on as usual.

3. Helping your child solve a weight problem will make her feel better—not worse. "Nobody would sit with me on the bus." "My gym teacher told me I was too slow." "I know I'll never get a date to the prom." Growing up is tough—and being overweight makes it that much tougher. Kids can be mean, peer pressure fierce, and a child's self-esteem can be quickly depleted by a few offhand remarks, careless gestures, or missed social opportunities. As a parent, you want more than anything to raise a happy, healthy son or daughter. So when your child makes comments like these, you listen. And you worry.

Does my child realize she has a weight problem? Will talking about overweight with my daughter make her self-conscious? Believe me, if your child is overweight, she knows it. And it is far better to help her solve the problem than to ignore it.

Your child's self-esteem depends in large part on successful social development. But overweight kids often have a hard time making friends and joining in. I remember one Fourth of July when I went to the beach and watched a pretty little girl who was overweight. As she played with her mother in the sand and in the water, other children her age ran around nearby, laughing and splashing together until the afternoon games started. A crowd of kids gathered and the races began. Drawn by the excitement, the girl stood on the sidelines, expectant and eager, but obviously hesitant to participate. What I saw in her eyes was longing. She wanted to be part of things, but fear—of being slow, of being different, of being laughed at—held her back.

The social feedback your child receives every day at school, on the playground, and in the neighborhood is building his character just as the calcium he takes in is building bones. Overweight children face so many social challenges—teasing, discrimination, rejection. The humiliation of being "left out" on the playground or picked last for teams can really hurt. And the teasing an overweight child has to endure can make life truly miserable. These challenges lead to daily psychological stress that can interfere with academic learning and discourage children from doing things they might in fact enjoy.

Damage to a child's self-esteem can happen at an early age. As I see it, it is the emotional health risks of overweight that are the most serious. Far from robbing your child of self-confidence, dealing successfully with a childhood weight problem can actually build self-esteem. By helping your child to set weight management goals and then work slowly and steadily to meet them, you are helping her to feel good about herself and her achievement as well as improving her physical health. Your child, whom you love and adore and cherish, deserves to have a happy childhood.

4. You don't have to say no to all the foods your child likes—there is room for plenty of food and even snacks in the Can-Do Plan. The Can-Do Eating Plan accounts for your child's nutritional needs and plain old cravings by eliminating them: Scheduling snacks into the daily menu along with a satisfying breakfast, lunch, and dinner means kids will feel full; making sure those meals and snacks include foods kids love means kids will feel fulfilled.

Don't get the wrong idea—my program provides balanced nutrition, with the correct amounts of vitamins, minerals, protein, and carbohydrates your child needs to grow. The Can-Do Eating Plan controls calories, watches fat, and ensures good nutrition. But it's also fun. Ask any of the hundreds of children I have worked with over the past fifteen years, and they'll agree.

5. Your child will not "grow out of" his weight problem. Many parents take a wait-and-see approach with their child's overweight. They hope their chubby child will grow out of it, that "baby fat" will turn into muscle and their tater tot will become a football giant. Once a baby is walking, that roly-poly look should evolve over the next few years into a more proportional, contoured shape. If it doesn't, it's no longer baby fat—especially if your child is no longer a baby! Some parents wait years before they try to get help with their child's weight problem. Don't make the mistake of thinking your child will just shed baby fat on her own. It doesn't work that way. Consider these facts:

- Obesity that occurs in early childhood and persists throughout childhood becomes more difficult to treat as the child moves through adolescence and on into adulthood.
- The older the child, the less likely it is that he will outgrow obesity.

In fact, in my experience, overweight children do not usually "grow into" their weight without some change in eating or exercise habits. True, a four- or five-year-old who is chubby may grow to be an active child and slim down on her own. But a child whose weight problem has persisted for a few years is unlikely to slim down without some lifestyle changes. I don't recommend that you wait and see. The time to help is now, before she gets any older, before she gains another pound.

6. You can learn to make the right choices at the supermarket without feeling overwhelmed. It's a challenge to sort through the tens of thousands of products that promise healthful eating these days. For example, the yogurt section alone can be too much for a parent to make sense of: regular, lowfat, nonfat, fat-free, fruit on top, fruit on bottom, mixed-fruit, blended, traditional style, Swiss-style, custard-style, yogurt with sprinkles, yogurt with graham snacks, yogurt with granola, yogurt with crunch, yogurt with Jell-O Jigglers— every kind of yogurt imaginable. What's a poor parent to do? That's where the Product Guide which lists over 400 items (pages 115–134) can come in handy. Anything listed there is an appropriate choice. With this guide, and the menus for meals and snacks in chapter 6, you can become a confident shopper, making the right choices every time. And I'm not afraid to name names: You will know exactly which brands to buy.

Your Child's Health

There is another important reason why you should take steps now to bring your child's weight under control. Excess weight in childhood could become an adult-size problem with potentially life-threatening complications. Are there immediate risks to the health of a child who is obese? Research thus far is inconclusive, except for that on adolescents in whom obesity is associated with coronary artery disease. Some obese children have symptoms such as high blood pressure and high cholesterol that were once evident only in adults; still, the relation of these childhood conditions to adult disease is unknown. One thing we do know. *The longer a child is overweight, the more likely he or she is to become an overweight adult,* with all of the accompanying risk factors associated with adult obesity: heart disease, stroke, high blood pressure, diabetes, gall bladder disease, and certain types of cancer. For obese adults, there are other risks as well: respiratory problems, orthopedic disorders caused by strain on the joints, and complications during pregnancy. Don't put your child at risk for these adult health problems. The time to act is now.

When You've "Tried Everything"

Cutting Out Sweets

When it comes to calorie counting, sweets are usually the first to go. We all seem to forget that three square meals a day can also be a calorie extravaganza if we aren't careful. Limiting snacks and desserts is not enough. There are calories in everything your child eats. In fact, your child can become overweight without eating sweets at all. If you're like a lot of parents, you've found out the hard way that cutting out the cake, candy, and cookies may not be enough. If your child has remained overweight despite these efforts, then you need to do more.

The Fat-Free Fallacy

Maybe you're one of countless families who have been through it already: You've gone fat-free. You continue to shop nonfat, low-fat, and "lite." You've switched to skim milk, fat-free cookies and muffins, low-fat cheeses, and nonfat frozen yogurt. But it's not working. Your child's overweight continues. And you're frustrated.

Although food manufacturers would have you believe that "nonfat" means "nonfattening," it just isn't so. Fat-free does not mean calorie-free. Plenty of my patients have come in complaining that they gained weight even after giving up fats for good. Too many calories from fat-free bagels and fat-free cookies is still too many calories. You can gain weight by overeating a low-fat diet. And so can your child.

Why Diets Don't Work

Traditional diets of any kind are doomed to failure when it comes to kids. On the advice of well-meaning friends, family members, or even the pediatrician, parents just like you continue to try to restrict their child's diet. Parents feel they must do something—anything—to get their child's weight under control. They have outlawed a specific kind of food ("no candy") or a specific behavior ("no eating between meals"), but it hasn't helped. Their child stays stuck in a body that weighs too much. By the time they come to me, they are frustrated and desperate. As one teenage patient joked, "I'm a Weight Watchers drop-out." They're out there—desperate "dieters" of all ages—wondering when, if ever, help will come their way.

Traditional weight-loss diets don't work for children because they:

• **emphasize the negative.** Anyone with an overweight child who has tried to enforce denial diets (no fat, no frills, no fun) knows how tough it can be. Most diet books—whether for children or adults—emphasize the negative. "Do not eat candy and desserts." "Avoid soft drinks." "Put away the sugar bowl."

"Quit eating 'junk' food." "Stop eating between meals." Children feel deprived—even when they're getting the calories they need—because they don't get any "kid food."

• **feel like a punishment.** With so many rules about what not to eat, an overweight child may feel he is being punished for his overweight. This feeling can lead to sneaking food or otherwise cheating on the diet.

• **create a yo-yo effect.** Weight goes down, weight goes up, weight goes down, weight goes up, in a pattern that continues for life. As you know if you've dieted yourself, rapid weight loss—the oft-promised "ten pounds in ten days" or even more than four or five pounds a month—may seem like success, but it usually results in this yo-yo effect.

A crash diet that lowers caloric intake dramatically is not a long-term solution. In a short time, this kind of diet actually changes the body's metabolism, but not for the better. Sure, you lose fast and you lose hard. But then, after your body has come to believe it needs less, you go back to your usual eating habits and weight gain quickly resumes.

• **take a steep emotional toll.** Few children have the willpower it takes to restrict the amount of food they're eating. For kids the idea of ice cream now is not connected with the prospect of weight gain later. The wrong kind of attempt at weight control can be as dangerous to the child as the excess weight itself. The pressure of trying, and the disappointment of failing, can be quite traumatic for a child.

• **make false promises.** A pre-teen or adolescent child in search of help with overweight is an easy target for a "miracle diet" advertising campaign; these approaches are full of false claims and put your child's health at risk. If you deny your child the opportunity to learn healthful eating now, he or she will inevitably turn to forms of dieting—the mixes, the powders, the fasting—that are bad news. They are ineffective in the long term, and they can be dangerous.

• **are not designed to meet kids' needs.** Adult diets are entirely wrong for kids, whose growing bodies have high nutritional requirements. Reducing caloric intake too severely could actually stunt your child's growth. When a child receives insufficient calories over time, his body uses whatever calories are available for essential functions, putting growth on the back burner. So excessive weight loss could actually keep your child's body from achieving its expected height.

 • **are almost universally hated by children.** It's a fact. Children hate diets. If an eating plan is too strict, your child might rebel against it by sneaking food in her room or stocking up on food by overeating at school, at a friend's house, or at a holiday gathering. And who can blame her? From a kid's point of view (and from most adults'), *diet* means *deprivation*: Give up desserts and snacks, give up butter and cheese, give up red meat—and often, give up enjoying a tasty and satisfying meal. Kids don't want to give up foods they enjoy any more than adults do—especially when their friends don't have to.

Why the CAN-DO Plan Is Different

The Can-Do Eating Plan is unlike any other program available for children.

 • It is designed specifically for children ages five through eighteen.
 • It includes foods kids like to eat—even snacks!
 • It allows children to socialize normally—day to day and on special occasions.
 • Kids love it.

They really do. "See, I *told* you I could eat that!" I've heard comments like this more times than I can count. When I first meet with a patient and his parents, I often get the sense that there has been some kind of battle going on. Fights erupt over what's for dinner, what the child can and cannot have, and whether or not he is "cooperating" with his parents' well-intentioned diet regimen. As one diet plan after another offers hope only to result in failure, the disappointment turns to frustration and anger on all sides. You blame your child. You blame yourself. Enough already! This program allows everybody to call a truce. When you commit to helping your child achieve and maintain an appropriate weight through the Can-Do Eating Plan, you can look forward to happier times almost right away. This simple plan is easy to follow and requires no special foods, complicated recipes, or extra effort in the kitchen. Because your child will be satisfied, he won't need to sneak food, overindulge at friends' houses, or pig out when the baby-sitter comes. He won't have to. The foods he enjoys will be part of his daily menu. He will learn what his choices are, and he will learn to control his weight.

FAST FACT: Pizza Pizza!

You can make any slice of pizza healthier by requesting half the usual amount of cheese and blotting off the oil.

Your local pizza parlor may serve much higher-calorie pizza than the national chains—up to 25 grams of fat and 631 calories per slice. But Domino's Pizza, for instance, reports less than 5 grams of fat and 172 calories per slice.

Pizza toppings have calories, too. In two slices of a 14-inch pizza, adding these toppings adds the following extra calories:

extra cheese	168 calories
bacon	135 calories
sausage	97 calories
pepperoni	80 calories
salami	57 calories
black olives	56 calories
ham	41 calories
onion	11 calories
green pepper	5 calories
fresh mushrooms	5 calories

Source: Tufts University Diet & Nutrition Letter, August 1994. *Environmental Nutrition*, February 1995.

Still, parents are understandably skeptical when they hear how flexible my eating plan is. They want what's best for their child, and to them that means a diet. "Why can he have this particular food?" "Is this snack really low in calories?" I've heard all these questions before. The Can-Do Eating Plan is not a fat-free plan, but many of the items I include *are* low in fat or fat-free. The fat content might be reduced, so the items have fewer calories. Or the portion size is smaller, which also helps control calorie intake. My plan calls for a balance of lowered fat and lowered calories at the same time. You don't need to worry about fat content: It's all done for you. So how does a bag of potato chips make it onto my "approved" list of foods your child can enjoy? The single-serving brand I recommend is only 90 calories. That's okay! Your child will be thrilled, and you can be too.

Ten Reasons Why You and Your Child Will Love the CAN-DO Plan

1. It's not a "starvation diet"—but a plan that includes three meals a day plus snacks.
2. Your child still gets to eat the things kids really like.
3. It's easy to follow—works just like a restaurant menu.
4. It's inexpensive—no special foods to purchase.
5. You can still serve normal family meals—no complicated recipes to follow, no extra cooking.
6. It eliminates family arguments and tension about food.
7. Your child can still have fun on holidays and special occasions.
8. There is no useless chart or recordkeeping.
9. The results can last a lifetime.
10. It works—You really Can-Do!

Kids don't want to be different from other kids. Especially in school, their big concern is feeling that they belong. What child wants to open a bag lunch filled with rye crisps and celery sticks? With this program, kids can eat the foods their classmates and friends are eating. They can avoid being teased about what they eat or how much lunch they pack. The Can-Do Eating Plan makes it easy for your child to socialize normally—at birthday parties, picnics, holidays, and the like—without feeling singled out because she's eating "special" foods. She can be just like everybody else. That's why she's more likely to stay with this plan than a diet.

Foods Kids Love

I think one of the reasons my patients have had such great success on my weight-control plan is that I understand what kinds of foods they want to eat. And I know that they really don't want to give up those kinds of foods. Recently, for example, a pediatrician referred a seven-year-old girl to me. At 85 pounds, Sarah was more than 40 percent above her ideal weight for height—by definition severely obese. She seemed frightened, sitting quietly as her mother and I discussed the Plan. When we worked out the program, Sarah's eyes lit up and she began to smile, clearly relieved. Later, her mother confirmed what I had seen. Before our session, she said, Sarah had been terrified, wondering what foods I was going to take away, how I was going to make her suffer in order to bring her weight in line. But the suffering ends when a child begins this program.

It's obvious why Sarah was afraid. Until now, diet plans for children have been scaled down versions of adult diets: A *handful* of melba toast, a *small* portion of flounder with lemon, a *half*-cup of cottage cheese—foods that taste bland to children,

---

FAST FACT: Candy Calorie Nightmare

A 1-pound box of Valentine chocolates contains 2,300 calories and 140 to 150 grams of fat.

Source: Tufts University Diet & Nutrition Letter, February 1994.

and will have them craving high-fat no-nos in no time. No kid wants to follow this type of diet. Not only are the portions small, but the food itself is adult food. What child voluntarily eats melba toast or filet of sole? Even the so-called kid-friendly snack suggestions show little imagination. Frozen fruit juice on a popsicle stick? There are many more appealing and convenient choices out there, and the Product Guide on pages 115–134 will show you exactly what to buy, listing more than four hundred brand-name foods that fit right into this flavorful eating plan.

The Exercise Connection

No eating plan will control weight without giving the excess calories somewhere to go. Of course, it may be easy to suggest that an overweight child get out there and burn off the fat playing sports or enjoying other activities, but it's not that simple. Just keeping up with peers can be a challenge for an overweight child. Imagine running up a flight of stairs with a 10-pound bag of groceries under each arm; that's what it would feel like if you, a full-grown adult, were 20 pounds overweight. You feel clumsy and slow, get winded much more quickly, and your muscles might ache from the strain. That's how an overweight child feels on the playground or in gym class. Sensitive about appearance, he might also shy away from the pool or the beach, dreading the possibility of wearing a bathing suit or removing a T-shirt. So encouraging more exercise doesn't always work.

Even for younger children, a few extra pounds can cause a huge strain. A 65-pound child with 5 pounds of excess weight has an extra 8 percent of body weight to deal with when she crawls across the monkey bars. Overweight children work their bodies harder than normal-weight children. Combine that with the feeling that their peers are laughing and pointing, and you can see why sports have little appeal.

But exercise is an important part of my program. As the weeks pass, you will see a difference in your child's activity level as weight normalizes and confidence grows. In time, your child will find the courage to participate in sports or play hard with the best of them. In finding that courage, children find themselves and recapture the pleasures of childhood. With luck, this interest in physical activity will become part of a permanently healthy lifestyle.

How the CAN-DO Plan Works

The Can-Do Eating Plan is simple: Select breakfast, lunch, dinner, and the recommended number of snacks from the restaurant-style menus in chapter 6. These menu plans and the Product Guide are your tools for success, offering your child an array of food choices for breakfast, lunch, dinner, and snacks. Whenever possible, I recommend snack items that are available in individual portions, which make calorie control easier for parents, and lunches and snack time more fun for kids. When "extras" come up—on school trips, after soccer practice, and so on—you'll learn how to factor these into your child's daily menu.

But weight loss is not the answer, at least not the complete answer. What we are after long-term is weight management by using a reasonable plan that makes it easy for your child to reach and maintain an ideal weight, through childhood and beyond. Successful weight management eliminates overweight over a period of months and years and keeps it off through continued sensible eating and regular exercise. Successful weight management is about all the things your child can eat, not the things she can't. Weight management is a natural way of living.

The Can-Do Eating Plan relies on informed goal setting to create an individualized program that works. There are no impossible promises—no "quick fixes." These claims are unrealistic and unhealthy. Crash diets and liquid diets have no place in the life of growing children, or even adolescents, who may seek out these programs on their own. Overweight young children, too, attempt to control their weight by secretly skipping meals, avoiding certain foods, trying to correct the problem in their own uneducated way. But what they really need is advice, supervision, and support.

Your child's support system begins with your family doctor, who can help you to select the right program for your child and alert you to any special health concerns your child might have that you don't know about. From there, the rest is up to you and your child, who, together with the Can-Do Eating Plan, can embark on a life-changing program that is truly easy.

How to Use This Book

I want this book to serve as your own private consultation with me, an experienced nutritionist who understands your worries, fears, challenges, needs, and goals for your child. *The Can-Do Eating Plan for Overweight Kids and Teens* contains all you need to know to set in motion an eating program that really works—for your overweight child and for you as a parent. I want you to read it cover to cover, to know all that I want you to know about giving your son or daughter a happy, healthy childhood.

I'm sure you'll be tempted to flip to chapter 6 straight away, scanning the menus and Product Guide for surprises such as pudding (low-fat!) and cookies. Go ahead. But then turn back to the beginning and read about how you can make these products into a sensible plan.

As you begin this wonderful new phase in your family's life, keep a few things in mind. First, stay with it. This is not a six-week plan. Six-week plans don't work, as most adults who have seen their weight yo-yo on various diets can tell you. This is a way of life, with no time limit. Results will be slow and gradual. But kids are so comfortable with this Plan that they will not notice the time passing.

Second, don't worry. Becoming obsessed with ounces and pounds won't make them slip away any faster. Let it happen. If your child sticks to the Plan, it will work its magic in time. Believe me, you will start to see results before you know it. A day will come when your child suddenly looks slimmer, moves more easily, has more energy. You'll know it's working.

Third, weight loss may not be appropriate for your child. Success will mean different things to different children. For one child, it may mean staying at the same weight and growing in height. For another, it may mean gaining six or seven pounds a year instead of fifteen or twenty. For a fully grown adolescent or severely obese growing child, it may in fact mean weight loss. Consulting with your child's physician is an essential first step in determining the extent of your child's excess weight and selecting an appropriate calorie level.

If you follow this plan carefully, enlisting your child's commitment to the food choices and other tips included here, there is no health risk at all. And you will see your child blossom—really feel better, inside and out—as self-esteem builds and physical health improves. Your child really can control weight, look better and feel great! I've seen it hundreds of times, and it's far and away the best part of what I do.

2

Is It Just Baby Fat?
Recognizing a Weight Problem

"It's just baby fat. She'll grow out of it."

"He's just a big kid."

"I only feed her healthy foods. No junk."

"He must have a slow metabolism."

I've heard all kinds of explanations from well-meaning parents of overweight children. Parents say these things because they care. But when you come right down to it, there is probably only one reason your child is overweight: He is consuming more calories than his body needs.

In some ways, the body is a simple machine. It takes in fuel—protein, carbohydrates, and, yes, fat—and burns only as much as it needs to conduct its daily activities. For instance, a 77-pound child sitting on the sofa for 10 minutes burns about 9 calories; that same child playing basketball for 10 minutes burns 60 calories. The more the body moves around, the more fuel it burns. If bodies were cars, we would fill our tanks, burn fuel until the gauge said we needed more and then fill up again. But our bodies aren't cars: We get our fuel from the calories in food. If you take in more calories than you need, your body will store the excess "just in case." And that's the key to overweight: Extra calories are stored as fat.

Does this mean that the extra calories we take in come only

from foods that contain fat? No. Extra calories can come from fat, carbohydrates, or protein. We all know ice cream has calories. But so does fruit. So does chicken. So does a glass of juice. Sugar, found naturally or added, can make a product high-calorie—a twelve-ounce can of Coca-Cola, for instance, has 150 calories. But the same size serving of Mott's all-natural apple juice has 180 calories. Although both contain the same amount of fat—0 grams—you could gain weight from drinking too much of either one. *Excess calories cause overweight, no matter what they're made of, no matter where they come from.*

The Myths and Facts of Being Overweight

Wait a minute, you may be thinking. Extra weight may be a problem for adults, but children grow taller every year. Can't a child "grow into" his weight, like a tiny puppy grows into his large, ungainly paws? This is just one of the many myths about children and overweight. Unfortunately, it's exactly that, a myth. And when it comes to overweight, there are many myths indeed:

Myth: My child will grow out of it. How I wish this were true! But the fact is, many studies have proven that an overweight child is more likely to become an overweight adult. The statistics are quite sobering; here are some highlights:

• **Fact: Half of overweight youngsters remain overweight into adulthood.** In a forty-year study, almost half of children who were overweight at age nine and a half "matured into obese adults, many with health problems."
• **Fact: Odds are, an overweight adolescent may well become an obese adult.** "If childhood obesity is not corrected by age twelve," another study says, "the odds for becoming an obese adult are four to one. If the obesity persists through adolescence, these odds rise to twenty-eight to one."
• **Fact: The sooner your child's weight gets under control, the better.** "Fewer than 10 percent of obese infants become

obese adults," according to current research. "But the likelihood of becoming an obese adult jumps to 25 percent among obese preschoolers, 40 percent among obese seven-year-olds and 75 percent among obese teenagers."

CAUTION: It is dangerous to restrict the fat intake of a child under the age of two, no matter where that child lies on the growth percentile. I believe that age five is the earliest appropriate age to begin working on weight management.

• **Fact: Defeating overweight may be tough for kids, but it only gets harder as they reach adulthood.** Research shows that "children who stay overfat through adolescence only have a one in ten chance of ever attaining permanent weight loss as adults."

There is nothing cute about a chubby childhood, and as hard as it is to acknowledge that something must be done—now—to end the problem, it's really the only answer. The sooner you and your child take steps to gain control over calorie intake, the better the odds of changing the outcome for good. Correcting the problem in early childhood—starting at age five or six—is ideal. But correcting the problem in adolescence is equally important, because the longer a child remains obese, the more likely it is that that child will become an obese adult. The plain truth is that without some dietary and lifestyle changes many kids do not outgrow their baby fat. They may have done so once upon a time, when high-calorie foods were less plentiful and kids were more active, but not anymore. Even the most active of children spend hours in front of the television, the home computer, or video games. And the food most of us eat is prized for its convenience, not its nutritional value.

The Child at Risk of Future Overweight

What about the normal-weight child whose family history or lifestyle may put him or her at risk for overweight? It's not always possible to predict overweight before it happens. But certain risk factors exist:

- A sibling has a weight problem. (If you've picked up this book because of one child's problem, you might take a moment to decide whether a brother or sister might also develop a problem later.)
- One or more parents is obese, or has struggled with a weight problem, perhaps since childhood.
- You've noticed your child eating when bored.
- Your child does not participate in many physical activities, such as sports, outdoor play, or walking.

If you feel your child is at risk of becoming overweight, consult your pediatrician. And use the suggestions in this book for teaching your child to eat right and get the exercise he or she needs to balance the calories-in, calories-out equation.

Myth: There is no such thing as too much fresh, nutritious food. As long as he's not eating junk, my child can eat as much as he wants. Sound like too much of a good thing? Well, it is. Sadly, even children in families who eat only freshly prepared meals made from wholesome ingredients can become overweight.

• Fact: Too many calories lead to excessive weight gain, no matter what foods those calories come from. I think some of the increase in childhood obesity comes from misguided notions about nutrition. Since the 1980s, we've become health- and diet-conscious as a nation, which ought to be a step in the right direction. But thinking healthy has led to some unhealthy eating habits: Handing a child a box of fat-free fig newtons thinking they're healthful and can do no harm is a bad idea. The recommended serving size is two cookies. Two. That's 100 calories right there. And guess what? Two regular, fat-*included* fig newtons have 110 calories, so there's virtually no difference in the number of calories you're taking in. And excess calories make you gain weight, whether they come from a product that contains any fat or not.

Dairy products are another place we tend to go overboard. When it comes to healthy foods such as milk and cheese, parents tend to think that more is better. After all, these foods are a great source of nutrition, with plenty of calcium to build strong bones. I recall one grandfather telling me with pride that his grandson drank eight or nine glasses of milk a day—two and a half to three times more than he needed!

Sometimes, what seems healthy—a big, crunchy salad piled high with fresh vegetables—might become a high-calorie disaster by the time you add the croutons, bacon bits, and a few ladles full of creamy salad dressing. But we often overlook this and think we are doing our children's bodies a much bigger

---

FAST FACT: "Healthy" Cereals

Beware of healthy-sounding cereals—they may contain many more calories than you'd expect. A no-frills choice like Kellogg's Corn Flakes has just 110 calories in 1 cup. But consider these high-calorie breakfast choices:

Kellogg's Nutri-Grain with Almonds and Raisins	160 calories in 1 cup
Kellogg's Cracklin' Oat Bran	306 calories in 1 cup
Kellogg's Lowfat Granola (without raisins)	420 calories in 1 cup
Kellogg's Müeslix Apple and Almond Crunch	280 calories in 1 cup
Kellogg's Müeslix Raisin and Almond Crunch with Dates	303 calories in 1 cup
General Mills Nature Valley Lowfat Fruit Granola	318 calories in 1 cup

favor than we really are. A trip to the salad bar, which parents may see as a healthy alternative to a burger and fries, can surprise you with all sorts of hidden calories.

Parents know what's best for their children—sort of. But they make mistakes, despite their good intentions. For instance, Brian, one of my patients, would come home from third grade every afternoon to a beautiful tray of fresh fruit his mother had prepared. She carefully watched Brian's food intake, limiting his desserts to one a day, but allowed him to have as much fruit as he liked. What she didn't realize was that her little boy was consuming 500 calories' worth of bananas, apples, grapes, and oranges in one sitting! That's about one-third of his entire recommended calorie allotment for the day. It's not hard to do—and despite all the good vitamins and minerals fruit contains, providing this much is not necessarily good nutrition.

Don't Kid Yourself . . . There Are Calories In:

the peanut butter you lick off the knife
the food you eat right from the refrigerator
the finger foods passed at a party
the samples you try at a store
the candy you take from a candy dish
the leftovers you eat off someone else's plate
the vending machine item you eat on the run
the peanuts you eat on an airplane
foods tasted while cooking
foods eaten along with diet soda
foods eaten while everyone else is asleep
foods eaten while standing up
foods that don't taste very good
broken pieces of crackers and cookies

Myth: If my child were overeating, I would know it. In fact, he hardly has any appetite at all by dinnertime.

• **Fact: Unless you follow your child every minute of the day, you simply can't be aware of all he's taking in.** In an average day, your child might fix his own breakfast, pack his lunch, take the bus to school, eat at noon, come home to a three o'clock snack, and then eat dinner with the family. You might not know how much butter he puts on his toast, whether he licks a knife full of peanut butter as he prepares his sandwich, shares a friend's pack of mini-doughnuts at the bus stop, celebrates a classmate's birthday with cupcakes, "trades up" for a bologna and cheese sandwich at lunchtime, or digs into the ice cream before you get home from work. If he hardly eats any dinner, it may simply be because he's full. And if this has been your experience, you're not alone: Many parents have told me their overweight child eats very little at dinnertime.

As children get into their middle school and high school years, they're becoming more independent and parents have less of an idea of what they're eating and how much. Their busy lives—with clubs, athletics, and part-time jobs—mean they're eating away from home more often. Teaching your preteen or adolescent child to make good choices at home and away is your best approach.

The difficulty parents have in influencing their child's food intake heightens when the couple is divorced and eating styles vary between households. The eating habits of children who split their time between divorced parents are especially hard to keep track of. Oftentimes, one parent, concerned about a weight problem, makes an effort to limit calorie intake, while the other parent has an "anything-goes" attitude. Two-family households and those with extended families present a similar problem: Mom or Dad might be comfortable setting limits, but Grandma and

Grandpa want to see a "clean plate" or surprise the child with a sugary treat.

Even a child who wants to control his weight may have trouble remembering everything he eats in a day. Research shows that adults and children tend to overreport their consumption of foods they think are good for them, and to underreport those foods that are not: It's human nature. In my practice, I am interested in what kids report having eaten, but I also look at the scale: If we're moving toward a child's desired weight goal, that's great. If not, we have to try harder. That's the bottom line. The only thing that really counts is whether or not a child is gaining excessively. It's not about what Mom or Dad says he's eating, or even what he remembers having eaten. And it's not about eating the same amount as other kids his age, because that's just not a reliable indicator.

Myth: If a child doesn't eat any more than his friends or siblings, he's not overeating.

• **Fact: Not all overweight children eat more than their regular-weight counterparts.** Overeating—cramming down three pieces of cake in one sitting, devouring an entire bag of potato chips—is not a prerequisite for a weight problem. What looks like a "normal" diet can still consist of too many calories for a particular child's body.

• **Fact: All kids are different and have different caloric requirements.** Not all children of the same age or height need the same amount of food. The calories one child is able to burn off may "stick to the ribs" of another child. Why? A combination of reasons: Genetics, caloric needs, activity level. Probably all of us have adult friends who can eat whatever they want without gaining weight, or who indulge in dessert each time they crave it without the least sign of cellulite. We all have different makeups, but the solution to avoiding overweight is the same: Determining the right amount of calories we need to fuel our bodies, and adding enough regular activities to help burn excess fuel.

Myth: I've read about the obesity gene—if my child is overweight, it's genetic, so there's nothing I can do. Other people in our family have had weight problems, too. Your child's body is a one-of-a-kind machine. Sure, that machine may be inclined to store the fuel it doesn't need. But a family tendency to weigh too much is all the more reason to determine the proper amount of calories your child needs to be healthy.

• **Fact: Your child *can* learn to control a weight problem by making some simple changes in how he eats and how much he exercises.** A genetic tendency toward overweight is all the more reason to establish healthy habits—eating right, exercising regularly—right now, habits that will last beyond these growing years.

Myth: You don't need to listen to a child who expresses concern about overweight. After all, self-doubt is a natural part of growing up. "Mommy, am I fat?" "I need to go on a diet." "No one likes me because I'm so big." Even when your child's weight has you concerned, you may tend to downplay the problem when it comes up in conversation. But such offhand remarks speak volumes. Don't discount the things your child says about his body.

• **Fact: Some measure of self-doubt is to be expected from time to time, but a child who frequently touches on the subject of overweight may be asking for help.** You owe it to that child to give it to him. In fact, when you finally make some concrete plans to see a doctor or change his eating habits, your child may well act as though a huge burden has been lifted. I've seen this time and again. One eleven-year-old boy, hospitalized for abdominal pain, was referred to me by his doctor for consultation. The little boy was thrilled; at 210 pounds, he was severely obese, and he truly wanted help. A good way to test whether your child wants help is to offer it: If she responds enthusiastically, you can bet that the time is right. No child wants to be rejected. No child wants to be miserable. No child wants to be overweight.

Myth: Encouraging weight control could lead a child to develop an eating disorder. Anorexia nervosa (self-starvation) and bulimia (binge-and-purge syndrome) have received a great deal of press in recent years, which has helped parents to recognize these serious disorders and seek treatment for their children. Many parents avoid confronting their child's weight problem for fear of triggering one of these disorders. But anorexia and bulimia are emotional disorders, not merely dieting that has gotten out of control.

- **Fact: Eating disorders are not about needing to lose weight.** Our cultural ideal of thinness may drive young women to diet, but it does not cause them to develop eating disorders. Anorexia and bulimia are not simply weight control taken to the extreme, but the result of existing emotional problems— often accompanied by depression.

- **Fact: Eating disorders are caused by unresolved psychological conflicts in which food and weight become the focus.** As Martha Jablow writes in *The Parents' Guide to Eating Disorders and Obesity,* "Anorexia [and] bulimia are not solely about food, or weight, or body size, though they may appear to be on the surface. Eating disorders are about focusing on food as a means to control, survive, or cope with the multitude of psychological dilemmas that face adolescents and young adults. Eating disorders are about feelings, about forging an identity as a young person, about low self-esteem, [and] about emerging sexuality."

- **Fact: Appropriate weight management for a child who is overweight does not lead to an eating disorder.** Helping your child properly control his weight will improve his emotional and physical health.

Myth: My child is "big," but I am sure his body is just storing up extra calories for his growth spurt. If you notice that your preteen child is becoming overweight, you may assume it's preparation for the growth spurt. But it isn't.

• **Fact: Weight gain in excess of normal is not necessary for the adolescent growth spurt to begin.** Though weight gain accompanies growth at this stage, excess weight gain should not. A normal amount of weight gain prior to puberty is necessary to allow for growth. But the bodies of children about to enter the growth spurt do not require excess fat. If the growth curve shows excessive weight, then your child weighs too much.

What Is Normal Growth?

To understand what amount of weight gain is excessive, it is essential to understand normal growth and weight gain. Your child's growth has been tracked from the beginning. Re-

Patterns of Normal Growth		
AGE	INCREASE IN HEIGHT	CHANGE IN WEIGHT
Birth–1 year	10–12 inches	Birthweight doubles by 4–5 months; triples by 1 year
1–2 years	4–5½ inches/year	5–6 pounds/year
3–10 years	2–3 inches/year	5–7 pounds/year
Puberty: girls: 10–15 years	8–10 inches (total)	45–55 pounds (total)
boys: 11–16 years	11–13 inches (total)	50–60 pounds (total)

member all those visits to the doctor in your baby's first year? At each visit, your baby was weighed and measured, and the information was plotted onto a growth chart, a standard graph that documents your child's growth. As a part of each regular medical checkup, your child's measurements are updated. Using this chart, your health professional can determine whether your child is growing properly.

There are two periods of very rapid growth in the life of a child. The initial period takes place during the first year of life, when a child's weight doubles by four or five months of age and triples by one year. The second period of rapid growth is during the adolescent growth spurt. In between these ages, growth is slow, steady, and predictable.

Some babies are born large and others are born small, and it often takes up to two years for a child to settle into his or her expected growth channel or percentile. Thus, a baby who is large at birth might in time fall into an average growth channel: Carly, for example, weighed 8 pounds 14 ounces when she was born, placing her in the ninety-fifth percentile, but she settled into the fiftieth percentile by her second birthday.

Kids vary a lot in the way they grow: Of a hundred youngsters who fall within normal height and weight ranges, about 5 percent are much taller and heavier than the rest of the group and about 5 percent much shorter and thinner. A child whose growth pattern falls right in the middle is at the fiftieth percentile and is considered average. A child whose growth pattern falls along the lower part of the curve, say, the twenty-fifth percentile, is smaller or shorter than average but still normal. And a child at the upper end of the curve—at the seventy-fifth percentile—is above average.

Genetics play a big role in determining normal growth and weight gain for a particular child. But kids can surprise you: Billy's parents are both a little below average in height, but he takes after his tall Uncle Jim. Jenna's parents are average height, but Jenna herself resembles her short, slight Grandmother Rose. No matter who they look or grow like, children fall into a predictable pattern of growth at around age two.

What Is Normal Weight Gain?

As children grow and change, increases in height and weight should remain more or less in proportion to each other. A twenty-fifth percentile for height should mean a twenty-fifth percentile for weight. A sixty-fifth percentile weight should roughly correspond to the same percentile for height. Some variation occurs from time to time, but if your child is gaining weight along the expected channel, his height and weight should increase proportionately and remain proportional throughout his growing years.

Ideal, Overweight, or Obese?

Ideal weight is when a child's weight percentile is the same as his height percentile on standard growth charts. For example, the ideal weight for a child who is in the seventy-fifth percentile for height would be a weight that is in the seventy-fifth percentile.

Overweight is defined as up to 20 percent above ideal weight for height.

Obesity is defined as weighing 20 percent or more above ideal weight for height.

Severe obesity is defined as weighing 40 percent or more above ideal weight for height.

How Much Is Too Much?

When is weight gain a problem? When your child's gain moves significantly away from his established pattern. Daniel, for instance, grew along the twenty-fifth percentile for both height and weight until age seven. But by age twelve, though his height was still in the twenty-fifth percentile, his weight had jumped up to the ninetieth percentile. That is the kind of red flag a doctor recognizes. The growth curve is a valuable tool for monitoring your child's development and is worth discussing at every checkup.

Along the way, when do you need to be concerned about excess weight gain?

- When weight appears very much out of proportion to height.
- When weight gain "crosses percentiles" in an upward direction on the growth chart, while height follows the same percentile.
- When weight, plotted on the growth chart, is more than two or three percentile curves greater than height.

Take the guesswork out of it—ask your doctor during the medical visit you schedule before beginning this Plan.

Clueing in to a Problem

If you're still trying to decide whether to take further steps to correct an apparent weight problem, consider the following areas of your child's life:

Clothes and body image. Clothes are categorized by size, so even when the number of pounds gained month after month seems like nothing out of the ordinary for a growing child, the fact that her pants are soon too snug or her sweaters are too small will probably not escape you. If the school clothes you bought your child in September are too tight (though not necessarily too short) by December, you might want to think about having your child's rate of weight gain assessed. And if your child's gym or school uniform is a size or more larger than classmates of the same height, you can probably conclude that he or she is larger than average.

Style of dress may be influenced by overweight, as baggy clothes without waistbands become everyday wear, and nothing is tucked in, not even on special occasions. You definitely know something's up when your child refuses to be seen in shorts or a swimsuit, insisting on wearing a loose coverup or a large T-shirt at the pool or on the beach. When your child refuses to try on anything but sweatpants and huge conflicts erupt about shopping for clothes, you can no longer doubt it: Your child is overweight.

Physical activities. Another red flag for parents is when a child who once enjoyed participating in physical activities suddenly starts saying he doesn't like them anymore. She took dance for two years; now she wants to quit. He absolutely lived for soccer three years ago, but never even talks about it now. A young child enjoys the playground one season, then stops asking to go the next. Or a child may change activities altogether: She played basketball for the past few years, but now she's taking up painting. Or a child may not abandon a sport altogether, but may back off from its challenges, playing positions that don't require much movement, such as outfielder or catcher in softball, or goalie in soccer. These changes in interest may not be based solely on ability; as a child becomes overweight, activities he once enjoyed become difficult and unpleasant, so he withdraws. Again, imagine carrying around two 10-pound bags of groceries. Now, imagine trying to play soccer while carrying around that extra weight. Sports are hard on overweight kids, physically and emotionally. Not only are

---

Ten Ways to Tell if Your Child Has a Weight Problem

1. His doctor tells you so.
2. Your child complains about being teased about her size.
3. Your child's clothes seem to get too small too fast.
4. Shopping for clothes with your child is a nightmare.
5. Your child refuses to be seen in a bathing suit.
6. Your child's friendships are suddenly changing.
7. Your child withdraws from activities he previously enjoyed.
8. You find yourself referring to her as "big-boned" or "large."
9. You notice your child huffing and puffing after a simple task such as climbing a flight of stairs.
10. Your child tells you he thinks he's overweight.

other children likely to tease them, but overweight kids may become quite critical of themselves.

Social activities. Children are not all equally sociable, and some indeed prefer to spend time alone. But if your child's social life has changed dramatically—from playing with friends and attending social events such as birthday parties and school fairs or dances to sitting home alone, claiming no interest in companionship—overweight may be the cause. Children can be cruel, whether in the classroom, on the playground, or at the rec center. Not all children feel comfortable telling their parents that someone is making fun of them, but it may well be happening, causing a social withdrawal that is extremely harmful to self-esteem and overall emotional health. As a parent, it's your job to listen and watch for clues: Social interests are replaced by solitary ones. Your child makes statements such as "Alex won't play with me anymore" or "Rebecca doesn't want to be my friend." Of course, changing friendships are a part of life, but when the withdrawal is sudden, peer reaction to your child's overweight may be a factor.

How to Begin: The Medical Assessment

If you are reading this book, then you at least suspect your child is overweight. You may see yourself and your child in some of the scenarios I have described, but still not be sure if overweight is a problem. There is one sure way to determine whether your child weighs too much: a medical assessment.

In one medical visit, you can accomplish all of your objectives:

1. Assess your child's pattern of weight gain and overall health to determine whether there is in fact a problem.
2. Establish weight management goals.
3. Select an eating plan for your child from among the four calorie-range options in this book.

The assessment. I strongly urge you to make an appointment with your child's pediatrician or your family physician, who can confirm an overweight problem and offer support. This evaluation involves a simple examination—no lab tests, no high costs—that will give you the information you need to implement an effective eating plan. Remember, the health professional is there for the well-being of your child. Do not hesitate to ask questions about any concerns you might have about your child's health.

The medical visit is nothing to worry about—for you or your child. You may wish to talk with your child about the reason for the visit beforehand. (More often than not, I have found that overweight children look forward to getting help—they may even ask for it—so don't avoid the subject!)

The assessment is fairly simple, much like a regular checkup, and may include a combination of the following:

- weighing the child on the doctor's scale
- a "pinch" test (no, it doesn't hurt!) in which a fold of skin, usually on the underside of the arm, is measured with a caliper
- a simple estimation of body fat known as body mass index (or BMI), using your child's height and weight measurements
- plotting each year's weight gain and growth on a chart to compare it with national averages
- a discussion of physical fitness level—where things stand and how to help your child to begin getting into shape
- a conversation with parent and child about eating habits, attitude in school, and feelings about body image
- a review of the child's family medical history
- a blood pressure measurement

During this visit, you will want to ask a few questions. Here are some examples to get you started:

- How is my child's health overall?
- Is my child overweight?
- Is my child at risk for heart disease? High blood pressure? High cholesterol?
- Does he need to slow down his weight gain? To maintain current weight? To lose weight?
- How tall will my child be, based on the growth curve?
- Is my child's weight average? What does that mean?
- If my child is not considered overweight now, is she at risk of becoming overweight later?
- Are there any medical conditions that could interfere with normal metabolism?
- Is it okay for my child to increase his daily physical activity? How should he start?

Establishing a goal. Your doctor will help you to select one of the following weight-management goals for your child, depending on his or her age, height, and stage of growth:

- Slowdown: Decreasing the rate of weight gain.
- Weight maintenance: Staying at the current weight as the body grows taller.
- Weight loss: Losing excess pounds.

Choosing a calorie level. Once your goal is chosen, your doctor will choose an appropriate daily calorie level from among the four options in this plan: 1,500 calories, 1,800 calories, 2,100 calories, 2,500 calories.

Then, using the menus and Product Guide in chapter 6, you can begin right away. Because the foods in this program are not terribly different from the foods you might choose for your family already, there is no need to wait until after an approaching holiday or another high-calorie special occasion to start.

CAUTION: Don't just guess which weight goal might work for your child: A professional medical evaluation is essential. You can accomplish all you need to in a single medical visit, using this book as your guide.

Your Child Is Not Alone

With so much emphasis these days on health and fitness, it may be hard to believe that being overweight is all that common. But thousands of children share your child's problem, and the numbers are rising. "Obesity has become a major disease among children and adolescents," reports Dr. William Dietz, who examined the results of several extensive studies of Americans and weight. "During the decade and a half between surveys, the incidence of obesity for six- to eleven-year-old boys and girls increased by over 50 percent, and for teenagers by almost 40 percent. More youths are getting fat and fat youths are getting fatter." Taking action now can interrupt this trend, and promote a lifetime of healthier, happier living for your child.

Medical Visit Checklist

Before you begin this plan, consult your child's health professional. You can accomplish everything in a single medical visit, so don't miss this important step.

Your child's health professional will:

- determine whether your child has a weight problem
- decide which treatment goal is appropriate:
    slowdown
    weight maintenance
    weight loss

- select a daily calorie level:
    1,500 calories
    1,800 calories
    2,100 calories
    2,500 calories

- give your child the "Exercise Okay," discussing your child's current fitness level and recommending some appropriate physical activities

3

How Did This Happen?
The Causes of Childhood Weight Problems

After the school bus drops Jason off at his doorstep every afternoon, he fills a bowl with chips and watches television until dinnertime. His fellow fourth graders have begun to exclude him from playground games, saying he is "too slow" or "clumsy" to join in.

Chubby since she was a baby, Katie comes from a family of "big" people.

Meals at Joey's house are social events where everyone is expected to fill up.

Lucy always gets a lollipop to make her hurts go away, ice cream if she behaves during an outing, and a candy bar if she cooperates at the grocery store. When her pediatrician recently recommended she cut down on sweets to slow her weight gain, Lucy had a tantrum, insisting on her usual treats.

Each child is unique, and the amount of food and physical activity that keeps one child's growth in the normal range may cause another to gain too fast. It all comes down to a balanced equation: Calories in - calories out. When more calories are taken in than are used up, a person develops a weight problem: Parents, wishing only the best for their child, search for an answer, wondering how this could have happened to their child. Clinging to the many myths about childhood over-weight, they try to persuade themselves that this, too, shall pass. Each time they notice a stranger whispering about their child, each time a well-meaning relative offers some misguided advice about weight loss, each time their child comes home from school complaining that someone has teased her, parents wonder how this could have happened, and whether they are to blame.

Well, here's some good news. *Parental guilt can stop here.* Children develop weight problems for a variety of reasons, many of which are beyond the control of either the parent or the child. As recent studies have now proven, heredity plays a significant role in determining the way in which the body metabolizes, or "processes," food. What is enough food for one child may be too much for another—even within the same family. Personal eating habits—the child's own likes and dislikes, his choice of foods away from home—are another factor. Cultural and family food patterns also influence weight: An abundance of food is a tradition in many cultures and geographical regions, but the heavily laden butter-, cheese-, and meat-filled dishes the family treasures may take their toll on a child who is gaining weight too rapidly. Cultural background aside, the family's own eating patterns might include high-calorie processed foods, frequent dining out, plenty of sugary juices, or even just too much of the healthy stuff, all of which can contribute to overweight. Emotional issues may lead a child to seek comfort from food. Physical activity is another area parents of an overweight child must address, seeking the right balance of calories-in and calories-out to achieve an appropriate body weight.

Unfortunately, certain changes in the American lifestyle—the increase in the popularity of "sit-down" amusements such as computers, video games, and television; the easy availability of convenience foods and snacks; fast food at every corner; even the invention of portable phones and remote controls and the decline of street play and physical household chores—have added (literally) to the mix, increasing the rate of childhood obesity alarmingly. With many parents working outside the home, after-school supervision and limit-setting may be lacking, and a child stuck inside until Mom or Dad comes home may binge on high-calorie snacks out of boredom, with no chance to get outside to burn off the calories. Let's examine these factors in greater detail.

Genetics

If you want to be healthy, the saying goes, choose healthy parents. Indeed, genetics play a strong role in our overall health, in everything from allergies to heart disease. Obesity is no exception. Research shows that children with overweight parents are more likely to develop weight problems than children of normal-weight parents. In fact, youngsters raised in families in which one parent is obese have a 40 percent chance of becoming obese themselves. Double the number of obese parents, and you double the likelihood to a tragic 80 percent. And obese children, we know, usually grow into obese adults. By adolescence, an obese child has a 75 percent chance of becoming an obese adult.

FAST FACT: Frozen Dessert Bars

Häagen-Dazs offers both high-calorie and low-calorie frozen desserts:

Caramel Cone Explosion	330 calories
Triple Brownie Overload	320 calories
Piña Colada Bar	100 calories
Strawberry Daiquiri Bar	100 calories

The 100-calorie options meet Plan guidelines and are a refreshing treat in summertime or anytime.

It's true that "big" parents may follow unhealthy diets that promote excessive weight gain. But it may also be true that their genetic makeup makes them gain weight more easily than other people. You may have heard a friend say, "If I even look at ice cream, I gain weight!" That friend may not have been speaking literally, but the feeling she was expressing is all too familiar to many overweight people. I remember when one patient told me jokingly: "My body has a memory for fat." It's true: some individuals are genetically programmed to be good at storing food as fat because they require fewer calories to perform normal daily activities and maintain themselves. A person with a genetic predisposition toward obesity might have any of the following characteristics:

- a metabolism that more easily converts calories into fat
- a greater than usual capacity for the expansion of fat stores
- a slower than normal ability to burn fat
- absence of a normal appetite control mechanism

What does this mean for a susceptible person? A person at high risk for obesity has a harder time controlling weight: The calories come in, and while some are burned, many get converted to fat, which the body then stores. Those at high risk may actually burn fewer calories than other people during normal daily activity and exercise. In the face of the readily obtainable calories that confront us daily, it would be hard for a susceptible person not to gain extra pounds. Some body machines just need more careful preventive measures than others in order to maintain a healthy weight.

"Why me?" you might ask. "Why my child?" Here's a little history. Once upon a time, when our ancestors roamed the earth in search of their next meal, the ability to convert food into fat easily and store it well was an important trait for survival. The ability to pump in some extra "fuel" by gaining fat is an adaptive mechanism designed to protect us from leaner times, which were quite common in earlier days. A crop might fail, a herd might die, a castle might be plundered. There were routinely times of feast and times of famine. People who could easily store excess food were better protected from such disasters, and more likely to survive.

Today, however, most of us feast daily with no fear of famine. Even illness, which is now treated quickly and effectively, is unlikely to draw severely on our fat reserves. So those stores of fat are of little use, and they are hard to use up. Though it was once a health advantage to have an efficient metabolism that quickly converted extra calories into fat, it is now a liability. The adaptive mechanism developed over generations and passed down from grandparent to parent to child to ensure survival has become a health risk factor, one that could eventually threaten the life of an obese adult. It seems unfair, of course, that some children must pay in pounds for eating the same kinds of treats that youngsters born with "thin genes" can get away with. Still, genetics are only part of the weight-gain picture. Children of slim parents can become overweight, too. There is more to the story than just the "fat gene."

Eating Habits

Of course, the first thing most of us consider when we think about overweight is eating too much. Change the calories-in part of the equation, we theorize, and you solve the problem. But it's not that simple. Again, it's a question of balance: the right amount of fuel for that particular body engine's needs. But many children aren't reliable fuel customers. Why not? Because they eat for many different reasons, not just because they're hungry.

Many parents are surprised to learn that hunger isn't the only reason their children eat. In our fast-food culture, in which toddlers sing soda jingles and pizza parlors make house calls, food is a symbol of good times, diversion, and a sense of belonging. Chain eateries lure children to fat-filled "fun" meals with collect-'em-all toys and inviting playground equipment. Manufacturers market cereals shaped and flavored like tiny chocolate-chip cookies and miniature Rice Krispie Treats. Kids beg for high-fat, sugar-laced foods because we as a culture have told them these foods will make them feel better. They aren't yet sophisticated enough to recognize the "hard sell" of an advertising campaign.

When a child grows up in a home in which food seems to equal love (picture the stereotypical grandmother urging an already full child, "Eat! Eat!"), then eating becomes a comfort, a friend that child can always turn to, now and in adulthood.

Many well-intentioned parents find it hard to say no—even when a child is clearly overnourished. I've often heard: "Cheese and crackers are a good, wholesome snack. I let him have as much as he wants." "How can I deny my little girl? What if she's really hungry?" Let's face it. Saying no is much harder than saying yes, especially when it comes to a whining child. But parents must realize that even though a child cries, "I'm hungry!" it may not always be true. There are a lot of reasons children ask for food:

- A tired preschooler may ask for food to push back bedtime.
- A child who gets teased at school may drown his sadness in milk and cookies at home.
- A teenager struggling with homework may eat to procrastinate.
- A third-grader, bored as his mother looks after his baby sister, may eat during every television commercial.

Or a child might eat to soothe emotional stresses, such as

- switching to a new school
- the birth of a sibling
- feeling upset about parental arguing
- facing the trauma of a divorce in the family
- feeling nervous about a parent's remarriage
- worrying about an illness in the family

FAST FACT: We All Scream for Ice Cream

Hot fudge, caramel, and butterscotch are the most popular ice cream toppings. How do ice cream toppings compare when it comes to calories and fat?

Two tablespoons of fudge topping contain up to 140 calories and 6 grams of fat. Two tablespoons of caramel, butterscotch, or strawberry topping have the same number of calories, with only 1 gram of fat.

Using candy and cookies as a reward, bribe, pacifier, or remedy for boredom is a mistake most of us parents make—even me! Through custom and culture, we have used food to feel good. For adults and children alike, eating accompanies most social events, from baseball games to birthday parties. Adults probably get together for a meal more often than they get together for any other social occasion, so why wouldn't children do the same? Inevitably, there is pressure to eat, regardless of hunger, to be a part of the crowd. Accepting an offer of refreshments is part of being polite. We have one more bite, one more helping, one more plateful to please the hostess—even though we are full.

And that's the attitude that can get us—and our children—in trouble: We eat even when we aren't hungry. But the fact is, hunger is a distinct and uncomfortable sensation, and kids (and adults) can learn to tell it apart from other physical and emotional pangs. We *don't* have to eat to be polite, to pass the time, because we're lonely, or because we see a McDonald's commercial.

Sometimes, "I want cake and ice cream" really means "I want to have some fun." Reaching for a handful of chips on a weekend afternoon may just mean there's nothing else to do. A child may really crave a candy bar, but he is not necessarily hungry for it.

In the Land of Plenty

A century ago, food was not as plentiful as it is today. As recently as 1950, some 500 different foods were available at any one time. Today, there are 50,000 foods offered in the average supermarket. Obviously, the food supply was very different in generations past. For our grandparents and their parents, meals were made "from scratch," and dinner preparation could take an entire afternoon. Food storage was a challenge, and fresh fruits and vegetables were available only in season. Baked goods and candy were a special treat, and snack foods scarce. The highlight of a child's week might have been a scoop of homemade ice cream on a Sunday afternoon. But modern technological developments in the areas of food manufacturing, refrigeration, transportation, and use of preservatives have made a dramatic difference.

Today, so much food is available instantly: Open up a vacuum-pack, pop it in the microwave, squeeze out the premade sauce, and you're there. If you prefer, you can grab a burger and fries without even leaving your car; if you miss the first fast-food place, there's probably another one on the next corner. Vending machines—at gas stations, in schools, at work, in apartment buildings and dorms—vie for our attention with a blinding array of chips, cookies, and sodas.

Convenience has its appeal. Many two-parent households are also two-breadwinner households, with all the scheduling hassles that phrase implies. And single parents, too, struggle to save time. Teenagers, busy with extracurricular activities or part-time jobs, tend to grab a meal on the run, or fill up on soda and chips. We need convenience. But it's costing us in calories. I developed the Product Guide in chapter 6 to show you how to make the most of convenience foods so they work for, not against, your child.

Bigger and Bigger

Besides providing so many choices, the food industry has affected us in other ways, too. Portions are larger these days.

English muffins now come in sandwich-size as well as regular. Bakery muffins, once palm-size, are often as big as small cakes. Soft drinks—some with free refills—are sold in sizes large, larger, and larger still. And even fruits are grown larger than before, increasing the number of calories; peaches, once two and a half inches in diameter, are now almost five. Apples, oranges, and bananas are all bigger than ever. Kids sit on the sidelines at sports events, gulping 32-ounce bottles of juice or sports drinks.

People celebrate abundance. Larger portions are a part of that celebration. We are lucky that food is so plentiful and so readily available today. With so much at our disposal, we may forget to consider portion size. Kids need help figuring out what a reasonable portion is. The Product Guide on pages 115–134 takes portion size into account and offers a simple way to evaluate new products for possible inclusion on your list of acceptable snack alternatives.

About Physical Activity

A body has to move around to burn calories, and movement is often the missing element when it comes to overweight children. Take a moment to picture a child playing. Do you envision him running freely across a sunlit lawn? Climbing a jungle gym? Suiting up for team sports? Now picture *your* child playing. Is he settling down in front of the computer? Sprawling on the floor in front of the TV for a video game? If these are the kinds of things you imagine, you are far from alone. Times have changed, even recently, as more and more kids sit down when it comes time to play. Walking to school, a friend's house, or the store is quickly becoming a thing of the past. Children don't work as hard at their chores, thanks to labor-saving devices such as riding mowers, automatic car washes, and the like. Family-oriented physical activity seems on the wane as schedules get ever busier. And street play—gathering with other neighborhood kids for some after-school or after-dinner activities—has gone by the wayside, which I consider a great loss for our children. The increase in childhood obesity reflects this trend. Fewer kids engage in daily physical activity, so fewer calories are being burned.

When it comes to overweight, there are two physical activity factors to consider: (1) activity level: How much fuel-burning exercise regularly occurs?, and (2) degree of fitness: How efficient is the body machine that is burning this fuel? The fact is, each person's activity level and degree of fitness have a dramatic effect on how the body uses its fuel. Fit people burn more calories than unfit people—even at rest. Being physically fit means having a higher proportion of muscle tissue in relation to body fat. The more muscle, the better. Why? Because muscle tissue requires and burns more calories than fat-storing tissue. Develop more muscle, and your body machine becomes more efficient at burning up your calories-in. So even when genetic makeup puts your child at risk of overweight, increased physical fitness can help to change the equation.

American kids today are alarmingly sedentary—which means they sit around a lot. Though anyone who has ever tried to keep up with a boisterous five-year-old knows that children love to move, the sad truth is that kids tend to lose this love of motion somewhere between the ages of eight and eighteen. "Children with average athletic abilities increasingly begin to drop out of sports and games beginning at about age nine," says physician Ken Cooper, who coined the term "aerobics" and now heads the Cooper Institute for Aerobics Research in Dallas. The reason, he says, is that organized sports programs are too often highly competitive, and less athletic children believe they won't be able to keep up with their more physically skilled peers. By age thirteen, most boys, and an even greater number of girls, have stopped participating in organized athletics or any type of regular activity.

Sadly, gym class rarely fits the bill. Across the nation, budget-crunched school systems are cutting back and even eliminating physical education programs; Illinois is the only state that mandates daily physical education. Even when gym is scheduled at least three times a week, opportunities for the recommended thirty minutes of sustained aerobic activity are rare. You might think your child engages in physical activity during each gym class, but in fact he or she may be watching instructional basketball videos or waiting in line for one or two turns on a balance beam. Busy teachers with large classes are less likely to take special interest in any but the "star players," so the nonathlete loses confidence—and interest.

Cutbacks in gym classes means that kids have to get their physical exercise before and after school and on weekends. But instead of walking or biking to school, most children today ride the bus or get a lift with Mom or Dad. As part of the latchkey generation, they very likely return home to an empty house, instructed to stay safely indoors until the parents come home, often after dark. It's no wonder that children choose

---

FAST FACT: Beware of Bagels

Calorie-counter books list a bagel at 150 calories. But brands can vary. Compare these popular choices:

Lenders Sesame Bagel	2 ounces	150 calories
Au Bon Pain Sesame Bagel	5.5 ounces	425 calories
Dunkin Donuts Bagel	3 ounces	225 calories
Large storebought bagel	4–7 ounces	300–550 calories

Add toppings, and you add calories. For example:

2 Tb. cream cheese	114 calories
2 Tb. peanut butter	190 calories
2 Tb. butter	216 calories
2 Tb. jelly	104 calories

Sources: *Environmental Nutrition*, November 1994; *Tufts University Diet & Nutrition Letter*, December 1994, *The New York Times*.

television and video games over other recreational activities. The statistics are alarming: The average two- to five-year-old watches more than twenty-two hours of television per week; the typical six- to twelve-year-old, twenty hours. Not surprisingly, studies show the more television a child watches, the greater his or her likelihood of being overweight. Yet what choice do kids have? Without an emphasis on regular physical activity as something fun to do—a part of daily life—it's simply too easy to give in to the temptations of TV.

Fearing for their children's self-esteem, well-meaning parents are often overprotective of kids who are clumsy or nonathletic, allowing them to quit the soccer team or take art and drama instead of swimming lessons or karate. But there is usually just as great an opportunity to build self-esteem through mere participation in a sport as in attaining mastery. Whatever sport or activity your child undertakes should be fun. If it's not fun, look around for another activity to try, but keep searching! Your child may well thank you for it one day. (I'm reminded of David, a formerly obese young man who is now at college, participating for the first time in intramural sports. "I always assumed I was terrible at sports, so I never tried," he told me. "But I'm not that bad. And I'm having a good time.")

In any event, all kids need a certain amount of exercise, though few are getting enough. Only two-thirds of American children get the recommended level of exercise. For many, a lack of exercise is a family tradition: Fewer than 30 percent of mothers and fathers of first- through fourth-grade children are physically active.

What effect has this had on our nation's children? The dismal evidence is in:

- Only 32 percent of children ages six to seventeen meet minimum standards for cardiovascular (heart and lung) fitness, flexibility, and abdominal and upper-body strength—a sharp decline from 1981, when 43 percent of this country's children were in acceptable shape. Fifty-five percent of girls can't even do one chin-up!

- Children today—and not just the overweight—are displaying grown-up–style heart risk factors such as high cholesterol and high blood pressure, symptoms doctors used to associate only with middle-age adults.

There is so much more at stake than just the physical appearance our culture puts such emphasis on. Children with weak bodies that weigh too much in childhood are like ticking time bombs, creating the potential for a lifetime of serious health risks.

The Bottom Line

Your child's particular equation—calories-in, calories-out—is unique. No matter what her siblings, friends, or classmates are eating, if your child is overweight, she is consuming more calories than her body needs.

Recognizing how a weight problem happens requires more than understanding the genetic risks of obesity, the varying caloric requirements of different children, and the role exercise plays in utilizing calories. Parents must also examine their child's particular eating habits, considering the role food plays in his life and looking for ways to bring the foods he eats in line with the food he needs. Even if there is a history of overweight in your family, it is not doomed to repeat itself in your

---

FAST FACT: Fat Consumption and Overweight

Americans have decreased their fat consumption from 40 percent of calories in the 1960s to 34 percent in 1990. Yet 33 percent of the adult population is obese, up from about 25 percent of the population just fifteen years ago.

Source: Environmental Nutrition, January 1995.

child. The "fat gene" is a risk factor, not a life sentence. The heredity-exercise-food intake dynamic is a puzzle that you and your child *can* solve. Learning to balance the weight equation—the correct ratio of calories-in to calories-out—can provide your child with a life skill that will change things for good, offering help for the present and hope for a healthy future.

4

Keeping Your Expectations Realistic:

Making a Long-Term Commitment to Long-Term Results

You've recognized your child's problem. You've met with the physician. Now that you understand the situation, you want results.

I understand. To be honest, I would love to be able to offer an immediate solution. I would love to be able to say to my patients' worried parents: "The solution is simple. Just feed your child grapefruit three meals a day for two weeks, and your problem is solved." Or "Just avoid candy and junk for the month of July, and the trouble is over." Though we all wish there were an instant answer to weight control, there isn't. As with so many other aspects of child-rearing, when it comes to weight management, patience is a virtue.

As natural as it is to wish that your child's extra weight and all the problems that go with it would simply evaporate, it just isn't that simple. And unrealistic expectations—your own or your child's—will not help your child in making and maintaining the lifestyle changes that will make overweight a thing of the past. So in this chapter, we will talk about how to establish reasonable goals that are easy to live with.

So often, children behave like adults when it comes to weight management goals. Older kids especially want to lose a significant amount of weight by a particular date, such as the first day of camp or the last day of summer. They want to lose weight magically, with no visible changes in their lives. They want a miracle cure. Unfortunately, it doesn't work that way. At least not quite. There is no magic pill to cure a weight problem. Here is what you can say to your child: *Eat what you like, but less of it, exercise more, and your weight problem will solve itself.*

Sure, it takes time. The results won't be instant, no matter how hard you hope for immediate change. But it will work.

Straight Talk . . . Tell It Like It Is

When kids want something, they want it *now*. So it may sound like a tall order to try to get them to try something that can't work overnight. How do I do it?

I level with them. It's that simple. I tell them the truth about their overweight, and I promise them that, together, we can beat it, little by little. Once they come in and hear what I say, they're hooked. Here's what I tell them:

- It took time to get to this point, so it will take time to undo it.
- Instant weight loss only results in instant regain.
- Diets designed for adults could interfere with your growth.
- My plan has worked for hundreds of children and adolescents just like you.
- We are a team. Together, we can bring your weight under control.

I communicate these things to them individually. I let them know I understand the pain they have been going through. I let them know that it no longer has to be that way. I tell them that good things are in store for them now that they are working to get their weight under control. And I talk about how much better they will feel, and how much more comfortable they will become at doing the things they've wanted to do but have avoided because of overweight. Kids understand what I'm saying, and it's usually enough to get them interested.

Following this eating and exercise regimen will get you and your child the results you hope for. You'll be taking over my role as coach. Give your child the same messages I would give him: "It's okay. This will work. We're a team." And mean what you say. This may be the most important challenge you and your child have ever faced.

Motivating a child in need of weight management is a lot easier than you might think. Kids *want* to follow this program. They *want* their overweight to go away. They *want* help. Why? Because kids want to:

- fit in
- be invited to do what the other kids are doing
- wear what the other kids are wearing
- play sports as well as the other kids
- make friends
- be liked
- be accepted

These strong desires are what motivate children—not health concerns that may not surface until much later in life.

FAST FACT: Cost Comparison of Natural vs. Regular

Americans spend $2 billion a year in health-food stores. Are they getting their money's worth? Consider the following:

Fat-free Nabisco wheat crackers cost one-third less than Frookie, a similar product available at health-food stores.

Supermarket-brand quick oats cost one-half the price of health-food store brand organic oats.

Nabisco Fig Newtons cost two and a half times less than health-food store fig bars. (The fat content is similar, unless you're buying fat-free versions.)

Once they're ready to confront their weight, all kids need is a game plan that works. And that's what I give them. As long as they follow it, they succeed. I don't recommend making any kind of contract with your child or writing a list of specific goals. Agreeing to follow the plan is enough.

How do you raise the topic of weight management with your child? Try using the same no-obligation approach I suggest to the parents who call to consult with me: "The doctor (or a friend) gave me the name of a nutritionist who works with overweight kids. How about if we go see her and find out what she's about? Then, we can decide from there." You can suggest using this book in the same way: Tell your child how you heard about it, and ask your child whether he wants to take a look at it with you—no obligation, just a look.

Your Own Expectations

As a parent, you can help your child by keeping your own expectations realistic. Here is what *not* to expect from your child:

- an immediate change in clothing size
- sudden athletic prowess
- unprecedented popularity
- a rapidly declining interest in "junk" foods
- instant shedding of excess pounds

Your child will not become a different person simply by embarking on this program (though the hope this program offers is often enough to renew a sad child's enthusiasm for life). The plan won't work overnight. But you will start to see some small changes almost immediately, changes so heartwarming that they will be reward enough for your dedicated teamwork. Here are some of the things you *can* expect to see in your child, sometimes within weeks of beginning the plan:

- A *gradual* change in body appearance. Once she's on the plan, your child may seem to be suddenly taller, as she continues to grow while her weight gain slows.
- An increased interest in physical activity. A nonathlete may never become an athlete, but as some of the awkwardness of overweight diminishes and confidence builds, your child may develop interests he never had: walking places with friends, Rollerblading, signing up for tennis lessons. Your child may even rediscover past interests that overweight prevented him from pursuing.
- Improved self-esteem that makes it easier to seek out and enjoy friendship. Social relations experts say there is a direct connection between how a person feels on the inside (confident or shy; happy or depressed) and how others respond to that person, so it makes sense that a child who feels better about herself will have an easier time interacting with peers.
- More self-confidence. Mastering a weight problem becomes part of your child's success story, and the result is a more positive outlook on life, a valuable personal resource that can stay with your child forever.
- A new understanding of what food choices are best, when it's okay to enjoy a special treat, and how to manage the calories-in, calories-out equation.
- And yes, in time, a proper height-weight ratio. Plans may differ—some kids need to maintain the same weight as they get taller; some need to gain fewer pounds this year than they did last year; and some need to lose excess weight. But children who follow the right plan for their needs will, in time, achieve their ideal weight and learn to control it for life.

If you compare these achievements with the instant results most parents hope for, they are not that different. They just take a little longer to achieve. But the good news is that they can be maintained into adulthood—which is the best way to avoid the negative health effects associated with adult obesity.

Out of the Mouths of Babes

Still, adults seldom list "feel healthier" or "have more energy" among their weight-loss goals. And it's hard to get children to think any differently. Kids and adults basically want the same things. Compare these lists of goals. One list was written by forty-year-olds, and one list was written by kids:

Lose 10 pounds by Christmas.	Look skinny by the first day of school.
Fit into a size 8.	Stop wearing "extra-large" sizes.
Look good in a bathing suit.	Stop wearing a T-shirt on the beach.
Look better for my sister's wedding.	Lose 10 pounds by the prom.

Appearances count, and even young children are aware of this fact. So don't discourage your child's interest in looking better. It's only natural, and if it's a motivator, then so be it. But find a way to identify other goals as well. After all, looking good is really just a by-product of feeling good, and feeling good is all about becoming healthy. And that's the real reason to fight your child's overweight now!

CAN-DO Goals for Weight Control

Now, I would like to share with you what my goals are for your overweight child. After all, this book is your private consultation with me, so I think you are entitled to know what I expect you and your child to get from my program.

CAN-DO Goal No. 1: Prevent overeating *and* undereating. Finding the right calorie level for your child's needs is the way to accomplish this. Again, it's about balancing the calories-in, calories-out equation. A growing child needs food. Eating the right amount for your child's particular body allows his weight to fall into place. Undereating could reduce the body's metabolic rate and may affect growth.

CAN-DO **Goal No. 2: Maintain proper growth.** My eating plan offers plenty of food, with few real restrictions. It's not a nonfat diet. It's not a low-calorie diet. In fact, it's not even a diet! It is a plan for eating enough food to maintain normal growth.

CAN-DO **Goal No. 3: Maintain proper nutrition.** Restricting a healthy diet can lead to nutritional deficiencies, which deplete the body's reserves and can affect growth.

CAN-DO **Goal No. 4: Put an end to yo-yo dieting.** Such dieting is ineffective, unpleasant, and a waste of time! My goal is to set your child on the proper course for maintaining a normal weight so that yo-yo dieting does not become a part of her life.

CAN-DO **Goal No. 5: To help your child learn to be responsible for his own eating and weight management.** When he is very young, your child requires your close supervision to be sure he is eating the right foods. As in other areas of life, eating is something your child gains more autonomy over as he gets older. Until age seven or eight, your child will follow your guidance fairly closely: You will stock the pantry and refrigerator, and you may still pack your child's lunches. By age nine or ten, your child will begin making more independent food choices, perhaps buying a school lunch or after-school snack, or joining friends for fast food after sports practice, so you will have less and less of a say in what gets consumed. Gradually, your child will take more responsibility for his own nutrition at home and away from home. By the teen years, it should be primarily up to him. Your role as a parent is to keep the house stocked with the right foods, offer your support, and let him take it from there.

CAN-DO **Goal No. 6: Improve your child's lifestyle.** I want your child to show increased physical fitness. I want your child to have a better social life, with less isolation because of how she looks and feels. I want your child to be more interested in group activities, especially sports and other outdoor activities. I want your child to feel good about herself—with more self-esteem and an improved sense of well-being.

In short, I want to change your child's life. Together, we can do that. With this program, your child can learn to manage eating without Mom or Dad playing the role of the "food police." With each month of success comes another building block of self-confidence for your child.

What Should My Child Weigh?

I really can't tell you what your child's normal weight should be. It's a shifting target. Growth and change are part of childhood. Normal weight for a child at one point is different for that same child at a later point. Because every child is different, growth charts don't always tell the whole story for a particular child. What may be appropriate in springtime will no longer be applicable by fall. I have not included height and weight charts in this book because I believe you need to consult with your child's health professional before determining what is normal for your child. The doctor can plot your child's previous growth pattern and then anticipate what course of action to take with regard to weight management.

Weight goals should be individualized. A child who gained weight at a normal rate until a year ago might require just a year's slowdown before weight normalizes. A fully grown adolescent who gained weight rapidly during a time of stress might be able to lose the extra pounds and then have no trouble maintaining normal weight afterward. There are many, many variables, and each person's metabolism and medical history are different. There is no absolute formula for determining which child should slow down his gain, which child should gain nothing at all, and which child should lose weight.

Selecting a Weight Management Goal

Your child's doctor will work with you to select a weight management goal that fits your child's own unique history. There are three basic goals to choose from, and they apply for all ages, male and female. Your role is to provide your child with the product guide–approved foods she wants for mealtimes and snacks and to make sure she has plenty of opportunities for physical activity.

After reviewing your child's medical history and weight gain pattern, your child's medical professional can help you to select from among the following:

• **Slowdown:** This category is designed for the child who is still growing but needs to decrease his rate of weight gain— for example, a child who gained 12 to 15 pounds in one year may now have a goal of a 5-pound weight gain for the coming year. Overweight improves over time as height increases and weight gain slows. (To ensure continued normal growth, height and weight measurements should be taken every three months, rather than the usual once a year.)

• **Weight-maintenance:** Also for the growing child, the goal here is to maintain the current weight as the body gets taller. Even three to five months' growth may be enough to normalize weight for some children in this group. (Check height and weight measurements at one month, three months, six months, and one year.)

• **Weight-loss:** This category is designed for the full-grown adolescent, who will not get any taller and therefore needs to undergo a program of gradual weight loss. Weight loss should proceed slowly to ensure safety and a lasting effect. This goal is also appropriate for the severely obese youngster who is still growing. (In this category, closer monitoring is advised. I recommend a height and weight checkup every two weeks for the first six months, and then monthly.)

Ideally, leave the weigh-ins and clinical monitoring to a health professional such as a doctor's staff member or the school nurse, which will relieve some of the pressure on both parent and child. It's best if the weigh-in occurs on the same scale each time. These height and weight checkups do not need to be part of an actual doctor's appointment, so long as there is consistency and objectivity on the part of the outside person doing the measuring.

Selecting a Goal

GOAL	OBJECTIVE	FOR
Slowed weight gain	Gain weight at a slower rate while continuing to grow in height.	A growing child
Weight maintenance	Maintain weight at present level while continuing to grow in height.	A growing child
Weight loss	Loss of ½ to 1 pound a week	A fully grown adolescent A severely obese* growing child

*"Severely obese" is defined as weighing 40 percent more than ideal weight for height.

CAUTION: Do not choose for yourself which category your child belongs in. Your doctor possesses essential information about your child's medical history and must be consulted in order to ensure safety and effectiveness.

How Long Will It Take?

I know you want results instantly, but no appropriate plan
for children can work that way. As a pediatric nutritionist, I
am professionally trained to provide for the growth needs of
children, and my program makes the most of that training. I
am deeply committed to helping children achieve their full
height by giving them all the nutrition they need to grow. A
high-intensity, short-duration restrictive diet is *never* an appropriate plan for a child. Weight normalization cannot happen
overnight. After all, your child did not gain extra weight overnight. Following this plan for gradual lifestyle change is the
best way for your child to achieve ideal weight. It's important
for both you and your child to learn to think in terms of
months and years and to celebrate the many successes along
the way.

Because this is an eating plan and not a diet, there is no
time limit. I really don't believe in saying, "Lose X amount of
weight by X date." To do so only sets a child up for failure.
Instead, I advise you and your child to look at this plan as a
new way of eating; when you add the exercise component, it
will become a whole new way of living. It's not a diet, so there
is nothing temporary about it. It really can serve as a plan for
life.

The Rewards

A lot of parents ask me whether they should reward their
children with prizes for losing pounds or sticking with the plan
for a certain period of time. My short answer is no. Why? Because the rewards will present themselves—in the form of
more confidence; greater interest in life, more fun, more excitement, new friendships, and an overall improved sense of
well-being and happiness. That's quite a prize. Those little
changes along the way are the things kids talk about most
when I ask them what they're getting out of the program:

"I can wear jeans now instead of sweatpants, and I even tuck
    my shirt in!"
"I've been invited to lots of parties."
"Now, nobody calls me names."
"On Mother's Day, Grandma said I looked great!"

Believe me, these "throwaway lines" are like precious keep-
sakes when you're helping your overweight child.
    Of course, your compliments along the way will mean a lot.
Let your son know how proud you are of his effort. Focus on
your daughter's hard work and the great job she is doing. And
celebrating success is worthwhile. I suggest planning some special outings together to celebrate your child's ongoing commitment to the Plan: A family hike, a biking excursion, a
backyard camp-out with friends. But don't base these special
events on reaching goals; rather, make them an ongoing part
of your child's new healthy lifestyle.
    Over time, you'll see your child begin to blossom with hap-
piness. The main reason families come to me for help is because their child is unhappy at his current weight and wants
to enjoy life more. Your child's commitment to weight management is a commitment to improving his life. As overweight
decreases, your child will find new interests—karate, hiking,
tennis, who knows? And the pleasure of pursuing these activities is reward enough for staying with the Plan.
    Social life can be a sensitive subject, to be sure. But it's also
a crucial one. More than anything else, kids want to be accepted by their peers. They want and need friendships. As your
child progresses with this weight-control program, you will begin to hear about a new friend or two, an after-school activity
your child wants to sign up for, or even how your child wasn't
the last picked when kids were teaming up for a school project
or sports activity.
    Clothing is often a tough subject when it comes to an over-
weight child. Conflicts often arise during shopping expedi-
tions—over how nothing seems to fit, how the styles the child

likes are unavailable in her size, how each shopping trip inevitably ends in misery. Dressing "like everybody else" is a big deal for kids so it's no wonder shopping is frustrating under these conditions. After a few months on the Plan, you will notice a change as your child begins to express pleasure at her achievements:

> "I can easily buy stuff off the rack—the same styles as the other kids!"
>
> "My clothes don't cut into my skin like they used to. Everything was so tight before."
>
> "I can still wear the pants I bought for school last spring, and now it's December!"

These may seem like inconsequential statements, but they matter. Self-image is made up of both what's on the inside and what's on the outside, so don't discount your child's interest in his physical appearance. It's okay to care about making a good impression. And feeling better about his appearance may lead him to socialize more and participate in more physical activities!

Falling Off the Wagon

As adults who have dieted are aware, weight management can be a struggle. There will be easy days and hard days, successes and failures, ups and downs. This is why overall goals are important. If she "falls off the wagon," let your child know that tomorrow is another day. The plan does not end just because she ate a candy bar on the school bus. All is not lost because she sneaked a soft drink at a picnic. Talk about it, walk around the block together—emphasize that burning some extra calories can help deal with those extra calories she consumed.

"It's Never Too Late to Have a Happy Childhood"

You may have seen the button that features this slogan on the lapel of a childlike adult. But it's relevant here: By giving your child the tools for effective weight management, you are giving your child the opportunity for a happier childhood. Above all, this program will allow your overweight child the chance to lead a normal life. I want your child to have normal eating habits. I want your child to enjoy a normal social life, to eat at restaurants, and go to birthday parties and overnight camp and school fairs and anywhere else he desires. The Can-Do Eating Plan is not a life sentence. It is a program for living.

FAST FACT: Herbal Tea Dangers

Beware of herbal teas that claim to help you get rid of unwanted fat. Some of those teas contain herbs that can stimulate the heart, raise blood pressure, and act as laxatives or cathartics.

Source: Environmental Nutrition, July 1994.

5

The Plan for Eating

"So what'll it be? Popcorn, cookies, or chips?"

"Which would you like, cherry or grape Fruit-by-the-Foot? Or how about a chocolate mint granola bar?"

"Frozen yogurt or ice pops?"

As the parent of an overweight child, you may not remember a time when you felt good about offering these popular snacks. For your child's own good, you have kept the cupboard bare of tempting treats. But despite your best efforts, your child continues to have a weight problem, one that even the strictest diet has been unable to solve. Well, I have some good news: "Strict" isn't the answer. And neither is "diet." The answer can be found in these next three chapters, which detail my eating and exercise plan.

This is, for me, the most exciting part of this book: At last, I can introduce you and your child to the information that will change life as you know it, creating a firm basis for your child's health and happiness, now and in the future. As the parent of an overweight child, you are making a truly loving gesture in setting things right before your child becomes an obese adult. This program can work for your child, as it has worked for hundreds of other kids. It's time-tested, nutritionally sound and balanced, and fun to follow.

CAUTION: The Can-Do Eating Plan is intended for children from age five through adolescence.

This program is just for kids; it's not a scaled-down version of an adult diet. It includes a balance of treats and staples that kids find much more than merely tolerable: Most of them actually *like* being on the plan. I think your child will, too. The food tastes good, the plan is easy to follow, and it works. That's enough to make everybody happy.

That's right, everybody—including the rest of the family. This eating program contains no special meals, and there is no extra work involved. These foods will appeal to your whole family. Although there are a few adaptations (lite pancake syrup versus regular, for instance), there are no huge sacrifices. The child with the weight problem is not being singled out, and the family isn't asked to sacrifice.

This is a kid-friendly program. It lets kids be kids. It's easy to follow and hard to fail. Best of all, there is no need to wait. Once you've taken your child to the doctor, you can begin immediately! Before a vacation? During the holidays? No problem. There is a way to work within the structure of normal family life. So why wait?

If I sound like I'm leading a pep rally, it's because I am. I want you as a parent to feel excited about beginning this wonderful lifestyle change. I want you to look forward—not only to the success to come, but to the process that can transform your child's life. And I hope you will convey this same hopeful enthusiasm to your child. I never want parents to become food dictators who say, "Things are different now, and you can only have what's on this list." No child should have the feeling that this eating plan is something being done to him alone. Instead, it should be a family commitment, something that everyone is doing together.

The Can-Do Eating Plan is well-balanced, low in fat, and controlled in calories. This Plan is fun because the foods it includes are fun foods, the kinds kids like. But don't be alarmed: This is not a junk-food diet. Either the foods themselves contain less fat than similar items, or the quantity is limited so that there is no chance of excessive fat consumption. For example, some fruit snacks have no fat at all; a bag of potato chips or a packet of cookies does contain fat, but because the choices I offer come in such small servings, fat content is not a problem.

If cookies and chips don't sound like diet food, it's because the Can-Do Eating Plan is not a diet. It's a medically sound eating plan that helps overweight kids achieve and maintain their ideal body weight without denying them the fun foods of childhood.

A Little History

Back in my earliest days as a nutrition student, long before I was married, I had a lot of ideas about how I would raise my children. I would make my own baby food, and it would all be natural. My children would be well-nourished, healthy kids who never even thought about potato chips or greasy french fries. Once I had my own family, however, reality set in. Time was scarce, and even when I had the time to prepare wholesome, natural foods, my kids didn't always want them! They wanted Mom at the oven baking cookies, not at the cutting board chopping carrot sticks. As a busy nutritionist, I didn't always have a lot of time to do either, so I have been very grateful to find so many packaged foods that are good enough to make it onto my "approved" list.

Don't get me wrong. I love healthy foods, and I really enjoy giving them to my kids. I love seeing them pop fresh strawberries into their mouths one by one, or hearing them ask me to buy more apples. But the reality is kids want more than strawberries and apples. They want to be able to enjoy all the same foods other kids do. And this program lets them do that.

I have designed this plan to be easy to follow. Your child won't complain, because the choices are so varied and appealing. And you won't complain, because the meal suggestions offer normal, everyday menus that your whole family will enjoy. With the Product Guide as a backup, you can use this book as a daily handbook for feeding your child right.

Ode to the Grizzly Chomp

You may wonder how it dawned on me that simply eating smaller portions and selecting lower-calorie foods they like could help kids normalize their weight. The truth is, this whole thing started with the Grizzly Chomp.

A long while back, Hostess came out with a snack cake called the Grizzly Chomp—a small chocolate cupcake with chocolate icing and sprinkles, and a bite taken out of it by the grizzly bear on the package. It was your basic Hostess Cupcake—with a big piece removed. The Grizzly Chomp was a perfectly delicious cupcake, just a little smaller than average. When I told my young patients they could snack on a piece of fruit, but if they wanted, they could also have a Grizzly Chomp, they were ecstatic! I knew I was on to something, and began looking around for other things I could offer as an alternative to the Grizzly Chomp. Over the years, many more products became available, and my list of favorites grew into the Product Guide in this book. Sadly, the Grizzly Chomp is history, but there are so many other choices these days that my patients don't even miss it.

You Mean My Child Can Have Sugar?

You bet. In fact, sugar is naturally found in children's diets from the day they are born. Breast milk is 7 to 8 percent milk sugar, or lactose. Studies have shown that babies prefer sugary substances from birth. This preference may have originated as a selective advantage: When our ancestors were still nomadic,

gathering nuts and berries, things that tasted sweet were probably safe, whereas things that tasted sour or bitter might have
been poisonous. While it is true we have far less need to live
by our instincts in this way today, there is no reason to ignore
this inborn preference. After all, even natural foods are high
in sugar. One-third of the calories in an apple, for instance,
come from fruit sugar, also known as fructose.

Honey, raisins, dried fruits, even fresh fruits and juices contain sugars that are no better or worse for the body than the
refined sugar in a typical candy bar, though the fruit and juice
have more overall nutritional value. But when it comes to
sugar—natural or refined—the body doesn't know the difference. So I have no problem allowing kids to enjoy sugars. The
trick is moderation: give a little here, restrict a little there;
make sure the overall nutrition is good, and the calories-in,
calories-out equation will balance out. When it comes to your
child, there is no reason to factor suffering and deprivation
into the equation.

"But sugar—especially from candy and sweets—makes my
kids hyper!" I have often heard comments like this one from
parents. Indeed, many parents are convinced that refined
sugar—the kind found in sweets—can cause children to become hyperactive, difficult to control, unmanageable, and
unfocused. They call it a "sugar high" and equate it to an
amphetamine rush; some even claim sugar is addictive, a claim
that research has proven false. Here's the truth: There is no
scientific evidence that sugar induces hyperactivity or other

---

FAST FACT: Hold the Mayo—Use Yogurt Instead

If you substitute ½ cup plain yogurt for the same amount of mayonnaise in a recipe for, say, chicken salad, you'll save 736 calories and
89 grams of fat.

disruptive behavior in children. In fact, a 1995 research paper published in the *Journal of the American Medical Association* analyzed twenty-three studies on the effects of sugar on children's behavior and found that sugar has *no* effect on children's behavior. The question remains, they wrote, as to why the study results differ so much from parents' impressions.

Let me offer some insight. There are many reasons why children might seem to go wild when they consume sugar.

- **Kids get excited when**

    —a special friend comes over to play
    —guests are arriving and there's an air of excitement in the household
    —it's the day of a birthday party (even before the cake and ice cream)
    —holidays are near (Halloween and other holidays are hyped for weeks, so kids are likely to get into the spirit. It's hard not to get excited.)
    —they receive a sugary treat not usually allowed

- **Some times of day may be more "hyper" for your child than others.** There may be a pattern—after school's out, when Mommy or Daddy comes home from work, after a nap, around bedtime. All of these are times when, coincidentally, you may give your child a sugary snack.
- **Behavioral problems may be blamed on sugar when there really is another cause.** Contrary to what many parents and teachers believe, behavioral problems such as acting up in class, not following rules, running around after being told to sit down, poor concentration, inability to complete an assignment, and being easily distracted are not caused by sugar.

The bottom line: When you expect your child's behavior to change after eating sugar, it sometimes does. But the fact is, kids just play hard sometimes. They get excited. That's how they are. It is a mistake to attribute such behavior to specific foods. I was at a six-year-old's birthday party last week and saw a dozen kids running around the yard, literally screaming with delight—and they hadn't had any cake or ice cream yet. Kids get physical, and they act out what they like, whether it's the latest action figures of today or the G. I. Joe of earlier generations. They are just playing. That's how they learn. My daughter's kindergarten teacher, now retired, commented recently: "Nothing has changed in thirty years. Banning action figures in school won't change kids' behavior."

And neither will banning sugar from their diets.

So yes, this eating plan does include some sugary snacks and other sweet foods. Why? In the words of Mary Poppins, "a spoonful of sugar helps the medicine go down." Include some sweets as Plan snack selections, and the results will amaze you:

- Your child will be more likely to stick to the plan if some sweets are included.
- Your child will feel more like part of the gang at school or with friends, and less like he or she is being punished or deprived because of being overweight.
- Your child will continue to enjoy childhood—or perhaps begin enjoying this part of childhood *guilt-free* for the first time in years!

This plan is very carefully conceived to provide balanced nutrition without excess calories. If you follow this plan, there are no risks at all to your child's health. If you can make your child happy with a couple of chocolate chip cookies at the end of lunch, by all means, do it. And feel good about it.

My Child Can Really Eat Fat?

Yes, and your child should eat *some* fat. A nonfat diet is never the right eating plan for a child, so my program is not fat-free.

My own scientific research on this subject, published in *The Journal of Pediatrics,* demonstrates that children need a certain amount of fat and cholesterol to grow properly. Furthermore, my colleagues and I found that it is actually dangerous to restrict dietary fat intake in children under two years of age— we found that limiting their fat intake hampered their growth and development. The American Academy of Pediatrics has issued the following guidelines for childhood fat intake: For children older than two, about one-third of the total daily calories should come from fat. Without that fat, they may not grow to their full height potential. This plan follows this critical guideline.

Adults have little need for fat in their diets and are healthiest when their fat intake is relatively low. But the adult of the species and the growing "cub" are really very different. Because children are growing, sometimes at quite a rapid rate, they need the high concentration of calories that fat provides. A newborn baby gets about 50 percent of his calories from fat for just that reason. Adolescence is another stage of rapid growth, as anyone with a teenager in the household knows. Generally, however, with fat as 30 percent of total caloric intake, a child can reach his or her expected size. To further restrict fat intake during the growing years of childhood is risky. Yes, there is a place for fat in a child's diet.

What Is Fat For?

Although dietary fat has a bad reputation these days, it does serve certain vital functions in the body.

- Fat is a carrier for fat-soluble vitamins A, D, and E.
- Fat prevents deficiencies of vitamins A, D, and E. A recent study suggests that those on low-fat diets may have trouble getting an adequate amount of vitamin E, which may be helpful in the prevention of heart disease.
- Fat from food is the only source for those fatty substances that the body cannot make itself.

So don't get suspicious when you see some high-fat foods on this plan—a few potato chips won't cause heart disease. But obesity can. And this Plan *can* help eliminate obesity. By correcting your child's overweight now through this plan of sensible, realistic eating, you are setting the stage for a future of health and well-being in which your child can enjoy food without overdoing it.

Our shared goal is to help your child to normalize his or her weight while achieving proper growth and development. My menus lower fat and cholesterol, but do not *eliminate* them altogether, because it's not necessary—and it's not healthy.

Doesn't Low-Fat Mean Low-Calorie?

The popular notion that eating an abundance of fat-free food will lead to weight control is false. *The New York Times* recently reported a study conducted at New York Hospital–Cornell Medical Center that proved this fact: Low fat does not necessarily mean low calorie. People can get fat not only on a high-fat diet, but on a diet high in carbohydrates, too. I for one am relieved that the world is finally realizing that fat-free is not the cure-all some once thought it was. Moderation is key: You cannot eat bowls full of pasta and gallons of fat-free ice cream and expect to control your weight. Fat-free binges are still binges. They are still caloric. They can still cause overweight. Excessive calories lead to weight gain. Period.

Author and physician Dean Ornish, M.D. claims you can *Eat More, Weigh Less.* Diet guru Susan Powter says "fat makes you fat." They both suggest you can load up on carbohydrates such as pasta and grains and still lose weight. Nutritionists are now saying that it's just not possible. "The idea that you can eat as much pasta as you want without gaining weight is patently ridiculous," says Marion Nestle, head of nutrition at New York University. "Calories are simply more concentrated in fat, but if you compensate for those calories from another source, it comes out the same."

Do fat-free versions of popular snacks and other foods have

a place in this Plan for Eating? They can. But fat-free does not mean calorie-free! Fat-free products have calories, too—sometimes an equal or larger number than the fat-laden versions of the same products. Parents often come to me saying they've tried everything—fat-free cookies, nonfat ice cream, nonfat milk—but their diet hasn't worked! When we total up the calories in all of those low- and no-fat foods, they far exceed the recommended numbers. So pay attention to what you're choosing. Better yet, let me choose for you by providing you with Can-Do menus and a Product Guide.

Otherwise, marketing hype may fool you. The best-selling cookie in 1994 was the SnackWell's fat-free Devil's Food Cookie. Total grams of fat? Zero. Total number of calories? 50. That's almost the same number of calories as a regular Oreo cookie, which is 53! So people consume more under the mistaken impression that they can do so without any consequence. After all, it's fat-free! These manufacturers are fooling some of us, but I bet that will start to change. Don't let a "fat-free" label be an invitation to gluttony. Fat-free does not mean "all-you-can-eat"! The solution? Monitor the calories, no matter what the food is. Or stop counting, and follow my Plan.

A Balanced Plan for Life

No matter which calorie level you will be working within, the Can-Do Eating Plan is completely balanced to provide proper nutrition for your child. That means all menus contain:

- About 50 to 55 percent of calories from carbohydrates (breads, cereals, grains, potatoes, rice, pastas, beans, fruits, and vegetables).
- About 30 percent of calories from fat (butter, margarine, oil, mayonnaise, cream, sour cream, cream cheese, and salad dressing).

- About 10 to 15 percent from protein (meat, fish, poultry, eggs, and dairy products).

The Plan also conforms to The National Cancer Institute's five-a-day guidelines by including five servings of fruits and vegetables daily.

Every day is already balanced. You don't need to count fat grams or calories. There's no math involved. I have done your

---

What Do Kids Really Need to Eat?

Children need to eat enough to have the energy required to grow and develop. They get their energy from calories. Calories are primarily derived from carbohydrates and fat. Carbohydrates, found in foods such as pastas, grains, breads, cereals, and fruits and vegetables, supply 4 calories per gram. Fats, from oils, butter, margarine, mayonnaise, cream, and salad dressings, supply 9 calories per gram, making them a more concentrated source of calories. Calories also come from protein (meat, poultry, fish, eggs, and dairy). Together, these foods also provide us with the vitamins and minerals essential for good health.

Caloric requirements vary with age:

birth to one year: 50 to 60 calories per pound per day
one to two years: 40 to 45 calories per pound per day
two to ten years: 25 to 35 calories per pound per day
ten to eighteen years: 30 to 40 calories per pound per day
adults: 15 calories per pound per day

For an overweight child, caloric requirements are calculated for ideal weight, not current weight. Other factors, such as rate of growth and activity level, play a role in determining appropriate individual calorie level. An active child burns more calories, so he may be able to consume more without gaining extra weight. Ask your doctor to determine your child's ideal weight and calorie needs.

homework for you. Just offer your child a selection from the menu that is part of a balanced day's nutrition.

Remember, your child's health professional knows best which plan is appropriate not only for your child's current weight, but also his or her age, sex, height, and growth pattern. Do not second-guess your doctor by putting your child on a lower calorie level than the doctor recommends. This will not help your child to lose weight more quickly, and may interfere with his growth.

Think about the four calorie levels your doctor will help you choose from: 1,500 calories, 1,800 calories, 2,100 calories, and 2,500 calories. You're probably amazed at these numbers. Does 2,500 sound like a diet? Of course not. The Can-Do Eating Plan is not a diet. It's an eating plan that works because your child will not feel deprived.

How can 2,500 calories be among the appropriate choices? Remember, not all overweight kids need to lose weight; some kids merely need to slow down their weight gain, and some are just trying to maintain their weight as they grow. Kids are not adults. They do not need to starve themselves on a thousand calories a day or less. A chubby seventh-grade boy will find himself ravenous as he shoots up like the proverbial beanpole once his hormones kick in and puberty works its magic. A growing child needs to eat. Just growing and developing burns calories.

Within each calorie level, your child will select from the menu as she would at a restaurant. Anything goes, as long as it's on our menu! If you're a label reader, you will notice that some of the foods on the menu have more fat than others. Don't let that worry you! If you follow the overall plan, the higher-fat and low- and nonfat choices balance out. This plan is nutritionally sound.

Eliminating fat and letting your child eat as much of everything else as he wishes won't work (as adult dieters who have tried already know). Selecting and adhering to the right calorie level is what will work—choosing lower-fat foods when possible and controlling portion size. And clearly, with 1,500 calories as the lowest-calorie Plan, no child will go hungry on the Can-Do Eating Plan.

Should I Read Every Label?

You can if you want to. But I've already done it for you. The Product Guide is the result of hours of label reading. I have included only those products that belong in our balanced program.

As for keeping a running tab on calories and fat grams, forget it. It's all been taken care of. Simply follow this Plan, and your child's fat intake will automatically fall within the appropriate range for that day, or for the week. There is room built in for school celebrations, after-sports snacks, and other unexpected events. With the overall Plan in place, things are bound to get much easier around your house—for you, your child, and the whole family.

Children Need Choices

Giving children the chance to say what they want is always important. I think it's one of the reasons I have had such phenomenal success in getting children to manage their weight and to maintain proper eating on into adulthood. My menus allow kids to select their own food each and every day— from a list of things they like, including treats that may have been forbidden to them before they started on this Plan. That's a real plus, because, especially with younger kids, control battles over food are common. Offering choices can help to alleviate the family tension that "Because I said so" can cause. Whether or not your child has a weight problem, it helps to ask, "Appetizer or dessert?" "Frozen yogurt or cookies?"

If children feel they are participating and being heard, they may sneak less food and will be more likely to control themselves when they aren't with you. Because there are so many

choices on each daily menu, this plan is painless, enabling you
to offer choices and seek your child's input on likes and dislikes.

When kids feel they are getting a fair shot, they feel better
about what you're asking them to do. Like you're in it together. Chapter 8 offers many suggestions for negotiation and
compromise. And as you begin the program, you will probably
find yourself turning to that chapter to aid in problem solving.
Ice cream after a school dance? No problem, but how about
skipping the evening snack that night? Pizza with the baseball
team? Great, but let's postpone tonight's dessert until tomorrow's snacktime. You'll get the hang of saying "Yes, but . . ."
quickly, and your whole family will appreciate the way it keeps
life running smoothly, without disappointment or upset. (In
time, your kids will propose solutions to you. Just the other
day, my six-year-old said, "Okay, Mom, I'll have this snack, and
that'll be it until dinnertime!" They will amaze you.) Being
overly rigid will backfire, so learn to compromise.

Isn't Snacking Between Meals a Bad Idea?

Forget about the "no eating between meals" rule some
adults follow to help shed pounds. Kids *need* to eat between
meals. They get hungry. And I'm glad to include between-meal
snacks that can stave off their hunger and keep them from
overdoing it when mealtime rolls around. I really believe in
the importance of snacking for kids. I think snacks might be
why they love this program so much.

How can kids snack and still control their weight? By selecting their snacks from the Product Guide. There are hundreds of choices, and many of them are sure to be among your
child's favorites! Yes, snacking is often where overweight kids
get into trouble. With so much available in stores, it's hard to
choose properly. But the trouble is over. All the kids on my
program get snacks—frequent snacks and *fun* snacks. So eliminate your child's worry right away, before you even begin this

program. Then watch the smile of relief spread across her face. It never fails—because snacking, or having to stop snacking, is what overweight kids worry most about!

Why Controlled Portions Are Important

Controlled portions are important because portions have gotten so out of control: everything today seems jumbo-size! So I am a big fan of portion control—establishing a preset amount of food that fits the needs of the calorie-level in question. Portion control is not only important at mealtimes, but also at snacktime. All of us tend to slide when we open up a half gallon of ice cream and start scooping; rarely do we stop at the half-cup serving listed on the package label. Individually packaged snacks take all the guesswork out of it. For this reason, I am a great believer in buying them. Sure, they may cost a little more, but they are worth it when you consider their benefits. With individually packaged snacks:

- You have fewer arguments with your child about how much is enough.
- You don't need to use a measuring cup or scale.
- You don't even need to read the nutrition information, provided the item is in the Product Guide! Any snack item offered there is an appropriate choice for your child.

I find that kids enjoy having their own personal pack. A single pop on a stick; a small bag of potato chips; a mini-size pack of Life Savers—these portion-controlled packs stop your child from going overboard. Check the Product Guide on pages 115–134 for acceptable choices.

What About Beverages?

A beverage has to have a flavor, right? Wrong. But any child you ask would probably agree that drinks should taste like something—orange, cherry, chocolate, berry. When kids are thirsty, that's what they drink. But flavorful drinks, even fruit juices, have calories. And some have more than you think. An 8-ounce glass of apple juice contains about 120 calories. The same amount of grape juice contains 170 calories. If you drink a glass of juice at breakfast, another at lunch, a few in the afternoon, one before dinner and one after, it would amount to more than 700 calories from juices alone in just one day! In fact, for some children I have worked with, cutting out juices and flavored drinks in their diets was enough to bring their weight into line.

You will notice that I don't include a lot of beverages on the Can-Do Eating Plan—not even fruit juices. The plan offers fresh fruit and some canned fruit snacks, but fruit juices appear only in small quantities. I don't recommend juices as a means of quenching thirst. If you can get your kids—whether overweight or not—in the habit of drinking water, you'll be ahead of the game. (If they balk at first, add a lemon or lime twist.) Try keeping a jug of water in the refrigerator. If you feel it will be too hard to ask your overweight child to drink water while your normal-weight child regularly helps himself to the gallon jug of cranberry-apple drink, then just switch to water for everyone! But don't feel you are depriving your family. Chances are, they drink more juice than they really need to.

If you're like most parents who've consulted me, you're probably thinking, Wait a minute. I thought juice was supposed to be good for you. It's better than a soda, right? A few decades of aggressive advertising campaigns have made most of us believe that drinking a nice, cold glass of juice is doing our bodies a favor. But glass after glass is just too much of a good thing, especially when overweight is an issue. As for bottled waters or seltzers, calorie-free is fine—but beware of flavored waters and seltzers, which contain "hidden" calories. As a rule, if it's not in the Product Guide, check the label for calorie content.

The Facts About Beverages

Beverages are a real source of hidden calories—and even the so-called healthy ones may contain calories. The labels require some detective work: Snapple lists calories for an 8-ounce serving even though the bottle contains 16 ounces. Arizona Iced Tea is usually sold in a 20-ounce bottle, bringing the count up to 237.5 calories if you consume the whole thing!

The best beverage choice? Aside from three glasses of bone-building skim milk a day, I recommend good old H$_2$O: Water is refreshing, thirst-quenching, inexpensive, and calorie-free!

BEVERAGES	CALORIES IN 8 OZ.	CALORIES IN 12-OZ. CAN/BOX	CALORIES IN 16-OZ. BOTTLE	CALORIES IN 20-OZ. BOTTLE
Snapple Fruit Punch			240	
Snapple Kiwi Strawberry			260	
Snapple Lemonade			220	
Snapple Grapeade			240	
Clearly Canadian Mountain Blackberry	100			
Mistic Mango Mania	110			
Ocean Spray CranGrape Juice	170			
Ocean Spray CranApple Juice	160			
Cranberry Juice Cocktail	140			
Hi-C Grape	130			
Arizona Iced Tea with Raspberry Flavor		150		237.5
Arizona Much Mango	100			
Pepsi-Cola		150		
Coca-Cola		150		
Cream soda		180		
Orange soda		210		
Black cherry soda		180		
Raspberry ginger ale		150		

BEVERAGES	CALORIES IN 8 OZ.	CALORIES IN 12-OZ. CAN/BOX	CALORIES IN 16-OZ. BOTTLE	CALORIES IN 20-OZ. BOTTLE
Ginger ale		135		
Grape soda		180		
Dr. Pepper		165		
Root beer		165		
Orangina	90			
Tropicana Fruit Punch	130			
Hawaiian Punch Fruit Juicy Red	120			
Grapefruit juice	100			
Apple juice	120			
Orange juice	110			
Prune juice	180			
V-8 juice	50			
Clamato	100			
Tomato juice	50			
Gatorade	50			
Tropicana Twister Orange Cranberry	130			
Juicy Juice Grape	130			
Welch's Grape Juice	170			
Hershey's Chocolate Low-fat Milk (2% milk)	200			
Hershey's Chocolate Milk (whole milk)	230			
Yoo Hoo	130			

The Good News

As you glance over the menus and Product Guide in the next chapter, you may be startled to discover something: Your child will be able to continue to eat pretty much the same foods he or she has always eaten! Maybe not the same amount of each, maybe not the exact same brand or recipe, but basically the same types of things. The food on this Plan is not diet food. It's real food, the kinds of things kids really like. Normal food, for normal kids. The only difference is that the calorie density is lower. For instance, you might select a Fruit Roll-Up for a snack that has only 50 calories, rather than a Snickers bar that has more than five times that amount.

Your child will enjoy a wide variety of everyday choices, made up of less-fattening foods. These are not unusual foods, nor are they difficult to prepare. They are the kinds of foods families usually eat. They are a wonderful surprise to children who are afraid of being deprived. The four calorie-level options are adequate to achieve goals and maintain growth and development; any extra calories that slip in unexpectedly can be burned up as your child increases her physical activity. So there's nothing to feel bad about, and more than four hundred things to feel great about.

About Artificial Sweeteners

None of the foods in this program contains Nutrasweet. Going sugar-free is not necessary. Your child can gain control of overweight without it. There are plenty of choices without turning to artificial sweeteners.

Aspartame, the chemical used in products like Nutrasweet, Equal, Spoonful, and Natrataste, is generally considered safe. There are more than 500 foods and beverages that contain it on the market today. But a number of side effects have been reported, among them headaches and heart palpitations. And who knows what researchers may discover later? Rather than wait until all the data are in, I chose to devise a plan using what I know will work without side effects: A carefully regulated selection of foods that contain sugar and fat, but in reduced amounts. With so many choices from among this category, the absence of Nutrasweet does not limit the choices in the least.

What About Salt?

If a child has normal blood pressure, salt intake is not a concern. If your child has high blood pressure—often caused by overweight—consult your child's doctor. Of course, moderation is advised in all things, so don't overdo it.

6

Get with the Program:
The Menus and The Product Guide

You're finally ready. You've been to the doctor, and you've established a weight-management goal for your child. So where do you start? Here, step by step, is how to proceed:

1. Sit down with your son or daughter and talk over the program. (See chapter 4 for some tips.) Explain that you will be using a set of daily menus and a Product Guide of approved brand names. Be sure to remind your child that this is not about deprivation: There will be plenty of snacks from day to day. Let your child know that there is room for flexibility when special occasions arise. And finally, talk about the role that physical activity must play to ensure the program's success.

2. Together, turn to your child's calorie-level menus. Your health professional has already helped you to select this level from among the four categories—1,500, 1,800, 2,100, and 2,500 calories per day.

3. Review the menus for breakfast, lunch, and dinner. Create a menu plan for the coming week that suits your child and the rest of the family.

4. Look over the snack section of the Product Guide to get snack ideas for the coming week. Note: Snack items are included at snack times *and* with lunch.

5. Together with your child, make a shopping list of the items you've selected.

6. Grab your shopping list, your Product Guide, and your child, and head for the grocery store to stock up on the items you've chosen. Most people shop regularly at a particular supermarket, because it's familiar and convenient. It's a good idea, though, to try a new store now and then, because you may discover products your usual store doesn't carry. Offering a variety of snacks and meal choices will prevent boredom. Be sure to look for single-serving packages to help with portion control.

7. Clear out the house. Don't hold on to any high-calorie temptations that haven't made the list. If you're afraid of "depriving" your other kids or your spouse, see chapter 8.

Tips for Success

- Establish regular mealtimes. Kids need structure, and a meal and snack schedule will make for better compliance with this eating plan.
- Don't skip meals. It can lead to excess hunger, which can in turn lead to excess eating.
- Making the right choices will be easier for your child if the right foods are available.
- If your child wishes, he may move an evening snack up to late afternoon on an especially hungry day. The evening snack is then eliminated for that day.
- If your child has an unexpected snack at school for a birthday celebration or at an after-school activity, consider suggesting that she forgo a scheduled afternoon or evening snack at home. Or find another way to balance the calories-in, calories-out equation, such as additional exercise or giving up a snack later that week.
- When you make unexpected changes, you need to negotiate and agree to them ahead of time. That way, there are no surprises, and your child will not feel angry or deprived later on.
- Don't nag your child. It only leads to resentment.

8. Emphasize choice: Let your child have as free a rein as possible for breakfast, lunch, and snack times. Dinner, however, is family time, so you can handle it as you usually do, following the menu suggestions listed here.

About the Daily Menus

The menus for each calorie level are basically the same; it's just the quantity of food and the number of snacks that vary.

CAN-DO **Breakfast**

Ask your child to select from this breakfast menu as he would in a restaurant. The breakfast items you have stocked up on, from among those listed in the Product Guide, are the choices available. Choose one selection from each category!

Don't let your child leave home without breakfast. When hunger is your enemy, breakfast is one of your greatest allies. A child who is ravenous by lunchtime will have a hard time staying within the expected limits.

CAN-DO **Lunch**

Everyone's hungry by lunchtime and ready for a break from the classroom. A bag lunch from home is the surest way to keep the lid on the calories. But no child looks forward to a weird "diet" lunch, so I've tried to keep things fairly normal on this lunch menu. The Product Guide offers brand-name guidance. If older kids have off-campus privileges for lunch, see chapter 9.

CAN-DO **Dinner**

It's cook's choice. I promised there would be no special foods to buy, no complicated recipes to follow, and I meant it: Dinner preparation can be similar to what you always do, with perhaps a few modifications in portion size and ingredients. But think healthy: No fried foods, please (try baking those potatoes instead of frying them!), and substitute low-fat cheeses for high-fat ones.

I want your child to eat less at dinner. Prepare less food so there are fewer leftovers, limit servings to first helpings only (no seconds or thirds) and avoid serving family-style, with heaping serving bowls of food set on the dinner table.

CAN-DO Snacks

Snacks are at the top of every kid's list of favorite foods, and it's what they worry most about giving up when they consider weight management. I see snacks as an essential part of this eating program, because kids find it helpful to have some "goodie" to look forward to. Your child will get snacks every day—and more than just one. Choices abound: a caramel-coated popcorn bar, a Rice Krispie Treat, a chocolate-vanilla twirl pudding, a few cookies, or any other selection listed in the Product Guide. The Can-Do Snacks menu for your child's calorie level tells what each snack time includes. Browse through the Product Guide to see what looks good.

Your snack guideline: Any item for 110 calories or less. But don't let the label fool you. For example, a snack-size pack of fig newtons is 100 calories per serving. But the number of servings listed is two, so the total calories per package is 200. *Check not only the calories per serving, but also the number of servings per package.*

Keep a variety of plan-approved snacks on hand so there are several options. And let your child choose his own snacks. Being able to select for themselves gives children a sense of freedom and eliminates the need for you to play "food police."

Through grade three or four, a midmorning snack is often part of the day, and I wouldn't think of taking that away. Either you'll pack the snack (in which case, use the Product Guide) or the school will offer a limited portion. This Plan assumes

When Is a Single-Serving Package a Calorie Trap?

I'm a big believer in individual packaging, but only when the contents fit into my plan. Don't assume that just any small pack makes it onto my approved list. When considering a mini-pack that isn't listed in my Product Guide, read the label for the number of servings in one container and the number of calories. If it's one serving at 110 calories or below, that's great.

But don't let individual packages like these fool you:

IN ONE LITTLE PACK OF	THERE ARE
Oreos	240 calories
Ritz Bits Peanut Butter Sandwiches	250 calories
Chips Ahoy! Cookies	200 calories
Cheez It Crackers	220 calories
Sunshine Vienna Fingers	280 calories
Wheat Thins	250 calories
Keebler Wheatables Crackers	170 calories

that a younger child may have a morning snack, so don't worry about having to modify the Plan.

For all children, the after-school snack is standard. It's also important: Kids are hungry after school, and they need this boost. The evening snack can be eaten right after dinner as dessert, or saved for later in the evening.

"I'm Thirsty!"

Beverages have far more calories than you think, so use caution. Juice, soda, bottled iced tea, fruit punch, sports drinks, flavored waters, lemonade—throughout the day, these can really add up. The Facts About Beverages chart (pages 82–83) shows how many calories can sneak in from beverages. Basically, I'm a big fan of plain old water—it's the most thirst-quenching and least caloric drink, and it's an essential nutrient for the body. Apart from water, I want your child to have three glasses of skim milk a day for protein and calcium as well as important vitamins. During meals and with snacks, your child may have the following:

Breakfast: 1 cup skim milk (One-half cup juice is among the fruit choices, but it is not a replacement for milk.)

Lunch: Water or 8 ounces Gatorade. Though I perfer that your child drink plain water; but some kids feel uneasy packing a bottle of water with their lunch. So I offer Gatorade only as a school-lunch option, because it is lower in calories than other drinks. (Beware: The sports bottle of Gatorade is 16 ounces, so it may be better to buy a smaller container than to ask your child to restrict himself to half a bottle.)

Dinner: 1 cup skim milk

Afternoon snack: 1 cup skim milk

The rest of the day, drink water.

These choices are fairly limited, and they may be somewhat difficult for your child to get used to at first, especially if he or she is accustomed to sugary drinks. Cleaning out the refrigerator and pantry of high-calorie beverages will make the transition easier.

By the way, if your child absolutely hates skim milk, 1 percent is okay. But I prefer skim.

Note: For all menus, calorie levels may vary up to 100 calories per day depending on your child's choices. All quantities are given in ounces (oz.) and standard measures: cups, teaspoons (tsp.), and tablespoons (Tb.).

What's a "small apple"?

In these days of giant-size servings, you may have to train yourself—and your child—to recognize when a piece of fruit passes muster. Fruit comes in a variety of sizes, but much of the produce available in the grocery store is large. Consult the following list for guidance:

FRUIT	SIZE	WEIGHT IN OUNCES*
apple	small (e.g., Macintosh)	4–5
	medium (e.g., Macoun)	6–7
	large (e.g., Delicious, Granny Smith)	8
orange	small (e.g., tangerine)	4–5
	medium (e.g., juice orange)	7–7½
	large (e.g., navel)	11–12
pear	medium	6–7
	large	9
peach	medium	6–7
	large	9
banana	small	4
	medium	6
	large	7 ½

*Weight includes skin, core, seeds, and rind.

THE MENUS

CALORIE LEVEL: 1,500

CAN-DO **Breakfast**

SELECT ONE

1 mini-box cereal, any selection from Kellogg's or General Mills variety packs or
   1 cup cereal of your choice from the Product Guide
1 Toaster Cake (corn, blueberry, raisin bran, strawberry, cinnamon apple, or
   banana nut)
1 frozen waffle (1 1/4 oz.) with 1 tablespoon lite syrup
1 SnackWell's cereal bar (blueberry, strawberry, apple cinnamon, or raspberry)
1 packet Quaker Instant Oatmeal (regular, peaches and cream, apples and cinnamon, blueberries and cream, or strawberries and cream)

SELECT ONE

1/2 cup apple juice	1 1/4 cups watermelon cubes
1/2 cup orange juice	1/2 banana
1 1/4 cups whole strawberries	1 medium peach
(or 3/4 cup cut strawberries)	1 small orange
3/4 cup blueberries	1 small apple
1 cup cantaloupe or honeydew cubes	

AND

1 cup skim milk

CAN-DO **Lunch**

1500

SELECT ONE

Turkey Sandwich: 3 oz. freshly roasted turkey breast, honey-roasted turkey, turkey salami, or turkey pastrami, on 2 slices 40-calorie bread with 1 tsp. mayonnaise (see Product Guide: Lunch Meats, pages 116–117, for additional choices)

Chef's Salad: 1 oz. turkey breast, 1 oz. lean ham, and 1 oz. low-fat cheese on a bed of mixed garden greens with 1 Tb. low-fat dressing and 2 4-in. bread-sticks

Tuna Salad Sandwich: 3 oz. water-packed tuna with 2 tsp. mayonnaise, served on 2 slices 40-calorie bread, 3-in. pita or 6 Saltine crackers

Yogurt: 8 oz. flavored, nonfat yogurt and 1 cup dry cereal of your choice (select either mini-box or see Product Guide: Cereals, page 115)

Ham and Cheese Sandwich: 2 oz. fresh, boiled, or baked ham (trim all visible fat) and 1 oz. low-fat American or Swiss cheese on 2 slices 40-calorie bread with mustard

Peanut Butter and Jelly Sandwich: 1 Tb. peanut butter and 2 tsp. jelly on 2 slices 40-calorie bread

Soup: 1½ cups homemade or canned chicken noodle, minestrone, vegetable, chicken rice, lentil, beef barley, chicken and stars, and 6 Saltines (see Product Guide: Soups, page 130, for additional choices)

Roast Beef Sandwich: 3 oz. lean roast beef (trim all visible fat) served on 2 slices of 40-calorie bread with 1 tsp. Russian dressing

Pizza: 1 slice (⅛ of 15-in. pie) regular cheese pizza (blot all the oil!)

SELECT ONE

1 small apple	12 fresh, sweet cherries
1 small pear	17 small grapes
1 medium peach	1 mini-box raisins
1 small nectarine	1 snack-pack diced peaches in lite syrup
2 tangerines	1 snack-pack mixed fruit in lite syrup
1 small orange	1 snack-pack pineapple tidbits in natural juice
2 small plums	1 snack-pack applesauce, unsweetened

SELECT ONE
1 bottle cold water
One 8-oz. box Gatorade (lemon-lime, grape, orange, iced tea cooler, watermelon, fruit punch, tropical burst, lemon-ice, citrus cooler, cherry rush, strawberry-kiwi, or cool-blue raspberry)

CAN-DO **Dinner**

SELECT ONE

Grilled Chicken Kebab: 3 oz. of grilled (or broiled) skinless chicken pieces, with tomato, sweet peppers, and onion on a skewer, served with 1 cup cooked rice

Baked Ziti: 1 cup casserole prepared with low-fat cheese and your favorite marinara sauce. Accompanied by 1 slice of crusty Italian bread and ½ cup tender string beans

Hamburger: 3 oz. ground round or sirloin on a lite (reduced calorie) bun, served with lettuce and tomato, along with ½ cup corn niblets

Salmon Teriyaki: 3 oz. of broiled or grilled salmon, served with 1 cup cooked bow-tie noodles and ½ cup steamed zucchini with 1 tsp. lite margarine

Chicken Fajitas: Two 6-in. diameter warm flour tortillas to wrap around 3 oz. marinated chicken strips, topped with chopped tomatoes, shredded lettuce, and mild or hot salsa

Broiled Loin Chop: 3 oz. tender lamb, pork, or veal chop, served with a small (4 oz.) baked potato with 1 Tb. fat-free sour cream, and ½ cup baby carrots with 1 tsp. butter and brown sugar

Spaghetti and Meatballs: 1 cup cooked spaghetti, prepared with your favorite marinara sauce and 1 medium (3 oz.) meatball, and a crisp garden salad with 1 Tb. low-fat dressing

Oriental Beef and Vegetables: 3 oz. thinly sliced sirloin stir-fried with a mix of crispy vegetables such as broccoli, asparagus, mushrooms, and sweet peppers. Served over 1 cup cooked rice

Arroz con Pollo: 1 cup cooked Spanish-style rice with 3 oz. chicken and ¼ cup tender peas

Linguine with White Clam Sauce: 1 cup cooked linguine and approximately 1/3 cup clam sauce accompanied by 1 slice unbuttered crusty bread and 1/2 cup Italian green beans

Roasted Chicken Breast: 3 oz. breast of chicken (remove skin after cooking), served with 1/2 cup mashed potatoes (prepared with 1 tsp. margarine or butter and 1 Tb. skim milk) and 1/2 cup freshly steamed broccoli

Pizza: slice 1/8 of 15-in. diameter pie regular cheese pizza (blot all the oil!), served with a small garden salad with 1 Tb. low-fat dressing

Asian Chicken Breast: 3 oz. grilled skinless chicken breast lightly brushed during cooking with hoisin sauce (available in Asian markets). Served with 1 cup thin noodles and 1/2 cup of mixed Oriental-style vegetables

Baked Cheese Lasagna: 3 in. square (made with low-fat ricotta and mozzarella cheeses), served with 1/2 cup steamed spinach and 1 slice unbuttered crusty bread

AND

1 cup skim milk

CAN-DO **Snacks**

The Product Guide contains an extensive listing of approved snacks from which to choose. Be sure to refer to the Guide for portion sizes.

AFTERNOON SNACK

This is an important snack, as most kids are very hungry after school. There's a long stretch from lunch until dinner, and kids will be eager for this one.

> ***CHOOSE ONE ITEM FROM THE SNACKS SECTION OF THE PRODUCT GUIDE, SUCH AS:***
> Strawberry String Thing
> Chocolate Chunk Kudos bar

One ½-oz. bag of cheddar cheese popcorn
1 Yoo-Hoo Fudge pop

SELECT ONE

1 small apple	½ banana
1 small orange	1 cup cantaloupe or honeydew cubes
1 small nectarine	1¼ cups watermelon cubes
1 medium peach	1¼ cups whole strawberries
2 tangerines	12 fresh, sweet cherries
1 small pear	17 small grapes
2 plums	1 mini-box raisins

AND
1 cup (8 oz.) skim milk

1500

EVENING SNACK
Lots of kids like to have something to "finish off" the meal. So the evening
snack can be eaten right after dinner as dessert or later in the evening.

CHOOSE ONE ITEM FROM THE SNACKS SECTION OF THE
PRODUCT GUIDE, SUCH AS:
Pop-Secret Popcorn Bar with Caramel Topping
Cherry Fruit Roll-up
chocolate pudding pack
One bag Doritos chips (9/16 oz.)

SELECT ONE

1 small apple	½ banana
1 small orange	1 cup cantaloupe or honeydew cubes
1 small nectarine	1¼ cups watermelon cubes
1 medium peach	1¼ cups whole strawberries
2 tangerines	12 fresh, sweet cherries
1 small pear	17 small grapes
2 plums	1 mini-box raisins

CALORIE LEVEL: 1,800

CAN-DO **Breakfast**

SELECT ONE

1 mini-box cereal, any selection from Kellogg's or General Mills variety packs or
   1 cup cereal of your choice from the Product Guide, pages 115–116
1 Toaster Cake (corn, blueberry, raisin bran, strawberry, cinnamon apple, or
   banana nut)
1 frozen waffle (1 1/4 oz.) with 1 Tb. lite syrup
1 SnackWell's cereal bar (blueberry, strawberry, raspberry, or apple cinnamon)
1 packet Quaker Instant Oatmeal (regular, peaches and cream, apples and cinnamon, blueberries and cream, or strawberries and cream)

SELECT ONE

1/2 cup apple juice   1 1/4 cups watermelon cubes
1/2 cup orange juice   1/2 banana
1 1/4 cups whole strawberries   1 medium peach
   (or 3/4 cup cut strawberries)   1 small orange
3/4 cup blueberries   1 small apple
1 cup cantaloupe or honeydew cubes

AND

1 cup skim milk

CAN-DO **Lunch**

SELECT ONE

Turkey Sandwich: *3 oz. freshly roasted turkey breast, honey-roasted turkey, turkey salami, or turkey pastrami, on 2 slices 40-calorie bread with 1 tsp. mayonnaise (see Product Guide: Lunch Meats, pages 116–117, for additional choices)*

Chef's Salad: *1 oz. turkey breast, 1 oz. lean ham, and 1 oz. low-fat cheese on a bed of mixed greens with 2 Tb. low-fat dressing and 2 4-in. breadsticks*

Tuna Salad Sandwich: *3 oz. water-packed tuna with 2 tsp. mayonnaise, served on 2 slices 40-calorie bread, one 3-in. pita, or 6 Saltine crackers*

Yogurt: *8 oz. flavored, nonfat yogurt and 1 cup dry cereal of your choice (select either mini-box or from the Product Guide: Cereals, page 115)*

Ham and Cheese Sandwich: *2 oz. fresh, boiled, or baked ham (trim all visible fat) and 1 oz. low-fat American or Swiss cheese on 2 slices 40-calorie bread and mustard*

Peanut Butter and Jelly Sandwich: *1 Tb. peanut butter and 2 tsp. jelly on 2 slices 40-calorie bread*

Soup: *1½ cups homemade or canned soup (chicken noodle, minestrone, vegetable, chicken rice, lentil, beef barley, chicken and stars) plus 6 Saltines (see Product Guide: Soups, page 133 for additional choices)*

Roast Beef Sandwich: *3 oz. lean roast beef (trimmed of all visible fat) served on 2 slices 40-calorie bread with 1 tsp. Russian dressing*

Pizza: *1 slice (⅛ of 15-in. regular cheese pizza pie [blot all the oil!])*

SELECT ONE

1 small apple	12 fresh, sweet cherries
1 small pear	17 small grapes
1 medium peach	1 mini-box raisins
1 small nectarine	1 snack-pack diced peaches in lite syrup
2 tangerines	1 snack-pack mixed fruit in lite syrup
1 small orange	1 snack-pack pineapple tidbits in natural juice
2 small plums	1 snack-pack applesauce, unsweetened

AND
1 snack from the Product Guide

SELECT ONE
1 bottle cold water
One 8-oz. box Gatorade (lemon-lime, grape, orange, iced tea cooler, watermelon, fruit punch, tropical burst, lemon-ice, citrus cooler, cherry rush, strawberry-kiwi, or cool-blue raspberry)

CAN-DO **Dinner**

SELECT ONE

Grilled Chicken Kebab: 4 oz. grilled (or broiled) skinless chicken pieces, with tomato, sweet peppers, and onion on a skewer, served over 1 cup cooked rice.

Baked Ziti: 1 1/4 cups casserole prepared with low-fat cheese and your favorite marinara sauce. Accompanied by 1 slice of crusty Italian bread and 1/2 cup tender string beans

Hamburger: 4 oz. ground round or sirloin on a lite (reduced calorie) bun, served with lettuce and tomato, along with 1/2 cup corn niblets

Salmon Teriyaki: 4 oz. of broiled or grilled salmon, served with 1 cup cooked bow-tie noodles and 1/2 cup steamed zucchini with 1 tsp. lite margarine

Chicken Fajitas: Two 6-in. warm flour tortillas to wrap around 4 oz. marinated chicken strips, topped with chopped tomatoes, shredded lettuce, and mild or hot salsa

Broiled Loin Chop: 4 oz. tender lamb, pork, or veal chop, served with a small (4 oz.) baked potato and 1 Tb. fat-free sour cream, and 1/2 cup baby carrots with 1 tsp. butter and brown sugar

Spaghetti and Meatballs: 1 cup cooked spaghetti, prepared with your favorite marinara sauce and 2 small (2 oz. each) meatballs, and a crisp garden salad with 1 Tb. low-fat dressing

Oriental Beef and Vegetables: 4 oz. thinly sliced sirloin stir-fried with a mix of crispy vegetables such as broccoli, asparagus, mushrooms, and sweet peppers, served over 1 cup cooked rice

Arroz con Pollo: 1 cup cooked Spanish-style rice with 4 oz. chicken and 1/4 cup peas

Linguine with White Clam Sauce: 1 cup cooked linguine with approximately 2/3 cup clam sauce accompanied by 1 slice crusty bread and 1/2 cup Italian green beans

Roasted Chicken Breast: 4 oz. breast of chicken (remove skin after cooking), served with 1/2 cup mashed potatoes (prepared with 1 tsp. margarine or butter and 1 tablespoon skim milk) and 1/2 cup steamed fresh broccoli

Pizza: 1 slice (1/8 of 15-in. regular pizza pie along with 1 topping [blot all the oil!]), accompanied by small garden salad with 1 Tb. low-fat dressing

Asian Chicken Breast: 4 oz. grilled skinless chicken breast lightly brushed during cooking with hoisin sauce (available in Asian markets), served with 1 cup cooked thin noodles and 1/2 cup of mixed Oriental-style vegetables

Baked Lasagna: 3 in. square (made with low-fat ricotta and mozzarella cheeses and lean ground beef), served with 1/2 cup steamed spinach and 1 slice of crusty unbuttered bread

AND

1 cup skim milk

CAN-DO **Snacks**

The Product Guide contains an extensive listing of approved snacks from which to choose. Be sure to refer to the Guide for portion sizes.

AFTERNOON SNACK

This is an important snack as most kids are very hungry after school. There's a long stretch from lunch until dinner, and kids will be eager for this one.

> *CHOOSE TWO ITEMS FROM THE SNACKS SECTION OF THE PRODUCT GUIDE, SUCH AS:*
> 1 bag of pretzels and a Nestle's Quik Ice Cream Pop
> Kudos, and nacho popcorn Cakes
> 1 Rice Krispies Treat and 1 raspberry Jell-O snack pack

SELECT ONE

1 small apple	1/2 banana
1 small orange	1 cup cantaloupe or honeydew
1 small nectarine	1 1/4 cups watermelon
1 medium peach	1 1/4 cups whole strawberries
2 tangerines	12 fresh sweet cherries
1 small pear	17 small grapes
2 plums	1 mini-box of raisins

AND

1 cup skim milk

EVENING SNACK

Lots of kids like to have something to "finish off" the meal. So the evening snack can be eaten right after dinner as dessert or later in the evening.

1800

CHOOSE ONE ITEM FROM THE SNACKS SECTION OF THE PRODUCT GUIDE, SUCH AS:

shortbread cookies
Flintstones Push-up Pop
one bag of Cheeze Doodles (5/8 oz.)
fudge dipped Granola Bar

SELECT ONE

1 small apple	1/2 banana
1 small orange	1 cup cantaloupe or honeydew cubes
1 small nectarine	1 1/4 cups watermelon cubes
1 medium peach	1 1/4 cups whole strawberries
2 tangerines	12 fresh, sweet cherries
1 small pear	17 small grapes
2 plums	1 mini-box of raisins

CALORIE LEVEL: 2,100

CAN-DO **Breakfast**

SELECT ONE

2 cups cereal of your choice from the Product Guide, pages 115–116

2 Toaster Cakes (corn, blueberry, raisin bran, strawberry, cinnamon apple, or banana nut)

2 frozen waffles (1¼ oz. each) with 2 Tb. lite syrup

1 Lenders Bagel (regular, not "Bagel Shop") with 1 Tb. cream cheese

1 egg, any style, plus 1 slice toast with 1 tsp. margarine

1 English muffin (sandwich size) with 2 tsp. jam

1 packet Quaker Instant Oatmeal (regular, peaches and cream, apples and cinnamon, blueberries and cream, or strawberries and cream) plus 1 slice toast with 1 tsp. jam

SELECT ONE

1 cup apple juice	1 cup applesauce
1 cup orange juice	1 cup fruit cocktail
1½ cups cut strawberries	1 cup canned pineapple tidbits
1½ cups blueberries	34 small grapes
1 banana	1 large pear
1 large apple	1 large peach

AND

1 cup skim milk

CAN-DO **Lunch**

SELECT ONE

Turkey Sandwich: *3 oz. freshly roasted turkey breast, honey-roasted turkey, turkey salami, or turkey pastrami, on 2 slices regular bread with 1 tsp. mayonnaise (see Product Guide: Lunch Meats, pages 116–117, for additional choices)*

Chef's Salad: *1 oz. turkey breast, 1 oz. lean ham, and 1 oz. low-fat cheese on a bed of mixed garden greens with 1 Tb. low-fat dressing and four 4-in. breadsticks*

Tuna Salad Sandwich: *3 oz. water-packed tuna with 2 tsp. mayonnaise, served on 2 slices regular bread, one 6-in. pita, or 12 Saltine crackers*

Ham and Cheese Sandwich: *2 oz. fresh, boiled, or baked ham (trim all visible fat) and 1 oz. low-fat American or Swiss cheese on 2 slices regular bread with mustard*

Peanut Butter and Jelly Sandwich: *1 Tb. peanut butter and 2 tsp. jelly on 2 slices regular bread*

Soup: *1½ cups homemade or canned soup (chicken noodle, minestrone, vegetable, chicken rice, lentil, beef barley, chicken and stars), plus 12 Saltines (see Product Guide: Soups, page 133, for additional choices)*

Roast Beef Sandwich: *3 oz. lean roast beef (trim all visible fat) served on 2 slices regular bread with 1 tsp. Russian dressing*

Pizza: *1 slice (4 × 4 in. square) Sicilian deep-dish pizza (blot all the oil!)*

SELECT ONE

1 small apple	12 fresh, sweet cherries
1 small pear	17 small grapes
1 medium peach	1 mini-box raisins
1 small nectarine	1 snack-pack diced peaches in lite syrup
2 tangerines	1 snack-pack mixed fruit in lite syrup
1 small orange	1 snack-pack pineapple tidbits in natural juices
2 small plums	1 snack-pack applesauce, unsweetened

2100

AND
1 snack from the Product Guide, pages 115–134

SELECT ONE
1 bottle cold water
*One 8-ounce box Gatorade (lemon-lime, grape, orange, iced tea cooler, water-
     melon, fruit punch, tropical burst, lemon-ice, citrus cooler, cherry rush, straw-
     berry kiwi, or cool-blue raspberry)*

CAN-DO **Dinner**

SELECT ONE

Grilled Chicken Kebab: *4 oz. of grilled (or broiled) skinless chicken pieces,
     with tomato, sweet peppers, and onion on a skewer, served over 1½ cups
     cooked rice.*

Baked Ziti: *1¼ cups casserole, prepared with low-fat cheese and your favorite
     marinara sauce. Accompanied by 1 slice unbuttered crusty Italian bread and
     ½ cup tender string beans*

Hamburger: *4 oz. ground round or sirloin on a regular bun, served with lettuce
     and tomato, along with ½ cup corn niblets*

Salmon Teriyaki: *4 oz. broiled or grilled salmon, served with 1½ cups cooked
     bow-tie noodles and ½ cup steamed zucchini with 1 tsp. lite margarine*

Chicken Fajitas: *Three 6-in. warm flour tortillas to wrap around 4 oz. marinated
     chicken strips, topped with chopped tomatoes, shredded lettuce, and mild or
     hot salsa*

Broiled Loin Chop: *4 oz. tender lamb, pork, or veal chop, served with a
     medium baked potato with 1 Tb. fat-free sour cream, and ½ cup baby carrots
     with 1 tsp. butter and brown sugar*

Spaghetti and Meatballs: *1½ cups cooked spaghetti, prepared with your
     favorite marinara sauce and 2 small (2 oz. each) meatballs and a crisp garden
     salad with 1 Tb. low-fat dressing*

2100

Oriental Beef and Vegetables: 4 oz. thinly sliced sirloin stir-fried with a mix of crispy vegetables such as broccoli, asparagus, mushrooms, and sweet peppers. Served over 1 1/2 cups cooked rice

Arroz con Pollo: 1 1/2 cups cooked Spanish-style rice with 4 oz. chicken and 1/4 cup tender peas

Linguine with White Clam Sauce: 1 1/2 cups cooked linguine with approximately 2/3 cup clam sauce accompanied by 1 slice unbuttered crusty bread and 1/2 cup Italian green beans

Roasted Chicken Breast: 4 oz. breast of chicken (remove skin after cooking), served with 1 cup mashed potatoes (prepared with 1 tsp. margarine or butter and 1 Tb. skim milk) and 1/2 cup steamed fresh broccoli

Pizza: 1 slice (4 × 4 in. square) Sicilian deep-dish pizza with 1 topping (blot all the oil!). Served with a small garden salad and 1 Tb. low-fat dressing

Asian Chicken Breast: 4 oz. grilled skinless chicken breast lightly brushed during cooking with hoisin sauce (available in Asian markets). Served with 1 1/2 cups cooked thin noodles and 1/2 cup mixed Oriental-style vegetables

Baked Lasagna: 3-in. square (made with low-fat ricotta and mozzarella cheeses and lean ground beef), served with 1/2 cup steamed spinach and 2 slices unbuttered crusty bread

AND

1 cup skim milk

CAN-DO **Snacks**

Your Product Guide contains an extensive listing of approved snacks from which to choose. Be sure to refer to this Guide for portion sizes.

AFTERNOON SNACK

This is an important snack as most kids are very hungry after school. There's a long stretch from lunch until dinner, and kids will be eager for this one.

**CHOOSE TWO ITEMS FROM THE SNACKS SECTION OF THE
PRODUCT GUIDE, SUCH AS:**

Honey nut Kudos, and chocolate chip cookies
Starburst Low-Fat Frozen Yogurt Cup and Choc. chip marshmallow munchie
1 bag of potato chips and grape Fruit by the Foot

SELECT ONE

1 small apple	½ banana
1 small orange	1 cup cantaloupe or honeydew cubes
1 small nectarine	1¼ cups watermelon cubes
1 medium peach	1¼ cups whole strawberries
2 tangerines	12 fresh, sweet cherries
1 small pear	17 small grapes
2 plums	1 mini-box of raisins

AND

1 cup skim milk

2100

EVENING SNACK

Lots of kids like to have something to "finish off" the meal. So the evening snack can be eaten right after dinner as dessert or later in the evening.

**CHOOSE TWO ITEMS FROM THE SNACKS SECTION OF THE
PRODUCT GUIDE, SUCH AS:**

Banana Crunch rice cakes and a Fudgsicle
Chewy Low Fat Granola Bar, Chocolate Mint, and vanilla-chocolate twirl
    pudding
Ritz Ark Animal crackers and a double fudge Brownie

SELECT ONE

1 small apple	½ banana
1 small orange	1 cup cantaloupe or honeydew cubes
1 small nectarine	1¼ cups watermelon cubes
1 medium peach	1¼ cups whole strawberries
2 tangerines	12 fresh, sweet cherries
1 small pear	17 small grapes
2 plums	1 mini-box of raisins

CALORIE LEVEL: 2,500

CAN-DO **Breakfast**

SELECT ONE

1 cup cereal of your choice from the Product Guide, pages 115–116, plus 1 slice toast with 1 tsp. butter or margarine

2 Toaster Cakes (corn, blueberry, raisin bran, strawberry, cinnamon apple, or banana nut) with 1 tsp. butter or margarine

2 frozen waffles (1 1/4 oz. each) with 2 Tb. lite syrup and 1 tsp. butter or margarine

1 Lenders Bagel (regular, not "Bagel Shop") with 2 Tb. cream cheese

1 egg, any style, plus 1 slice toast with 2 tsp. butter or margarine

1 English muffin (sandwich size) with 2 tsp. jam and 1 tsp. butter or margarine

1 packet Quaker Instant Oatmeal (regular, peaches and cream, apples and cinnamon, blueberries and cream, or strawberries and cream) plus 1 slice toast with 1 tsp. jam and 1 tsp. margarine or butter

SELECT ONE

1 cup apple juice	*1 cup applesauce*
1 cup orange juice	*1 cup fruit cocktail*
1 1/2 cups whole strawberries	*1 cup canned pineapple tidbits*
1 1/2 cups blueberries	*34 small grapes*
1 banana	*1 large pear*
1 large apple	*1 large peach*

AND

1 1/2 cups skim milk

CAN-DO **Lunch**

SELECT ONE

Turkey Sandwich: 3 oz. freshly roasted turkey breast, honey-roasted turkey, turkey salami, or turkey pastrami, on 2 slices regular bread with 2 tsp. mayonnaise (See Product Guide: Lunch Meats, pages 116–117, for additional choices)

Chef's Salad: 1 oz. turkey breast, 1 oz. lean ham, and 1 oz. low-fat cheese on a bed of mixed garden greens with 2 Tb. low-fat dressing and four 4-in. breadsticks

Tuna Salad Sandwich: 3 oz. water-packed tuna with 1 Tb. mayonnaise, served on 2 slices regular bread, one 6-in. pita, or 12 Saltines

Ham and Cheese Sandwich: 2 oz. fresh, boiled, or baked ham (trim all visible fat) and 1 oz. regular American or Swiss cheese on 2 slices regular bread with 1 tsp. mayonnaise

Peanut Butter and Jelly Sandwich: 1½ Tb. peanut butter and 2 tsp. jelly on 2 slices regular bread

Soup: 1½ cups homemade or canned soup (chicken noodle, minestrone, vegetable, chicken rice, lentil, beef barley, chicken and stars), plus 12 Saltines (see Product Guide: Soups, page 133, for additional choices), served with a crisp garden salad and 1 Tb. low-fat dressing

Roast Beef Sandwich: 3 oz. lean roast beef (trim all visible fat) on 2 slices regular bread with 1 Tb. Russian dressing

Pizza: 1 slice (4 × 4 in. square) Sicilian deep-dish pizza (blot all the oil!), served with a small salad with 1 Tb. low-fat dressing

SELECT ONE

1 small apple	12 fresh, sweet cherries
1 small pear	17 small grapes
1 medium peach	1 mini-box raisins
1 small nectarine	1 snack-pack diced peaches in lite syrup
2 tangerines	1 snack-pack mixed fruit in lite syrup
2 small plums	1 snack-pack pineapple tidbits in natural juice
1 small orange	1 snack-pack applesauce, unsweetened

2500

AND

1 snack from the snack list in the Product Guide

SELECT ONE

1 bottle cold water

One 8-ounce box Gatorade (lemon-lime, grape, orange, iced tea cooler, watermelon, fruit punch, tropical burst, lemon-ice, citrus cooler, cherry rush, strawberry-kiwi, or cool-blue raspberry)

CAN-DO **Dinner**

SELECT ONE

Grilled Chicken Kebab: 4 oz. grilled (or broiled) skinless chicken pieces, with tomato, sweet pepper, and onion on a skewer, served with 2 cups cooked rice and 1 tsp. butter or margarine

Baked Ziti: 2 cups casserole prepared with low-fat cheese and your favorite marinara sauce. Accompanied by 2 slices crusty Italian bread and ½ cup tender string beans and 1 tsp. butter or margarine

Hamburger: 4 oz. ground round or sirloin on a regular bun, served with lettuce and tomato, along with 1 cup corn niblets and 1 tsp. butter or margarine

Salmon Teriyaki: 4 oz. broiled or grilled salmon, served with 2 cups cooked bow-tie noodles and ½ cup steamed zucchini with 1 tsp. butter or margarine

Chicken Fajitas: Three 6-in. diameter warm flour tortillas to wrap around 4 oz. marinated chicken strips, topped with chopped tomatoes, shredded lettuce, ⅛ medium avocado, ⅓ cup pinto beans, and mild or hot salsa

Broiled Loin Chop: 4 oz. lamb, pork, or veal chop, served with a 6 oz. medium baked potato and 2 Tb. regular sour cream, ½ cup baby carrots with 1 tsp. butter and brown sugar and 1 small dinner roll

Spaghetti and Meatballs: 1 ½ cups cooked spaghetti, prepared with your favorite marinara sauce and 2 small (2 oz. each) meatballs, 1 slice crusty Italian bread with 1 tsp. margarine or butter, and a crisp garden salad with 1 Tb. low-fat dressing

Oriental Beef and Vegetables: 4 oz. thinly sliced sirloin stir-fried with a mix of crispy vegetables such as broccoli, asparagus, mushrooms, and sweet peppers, served over 2 cups cooked rice topped with 1 Tb. toasted sesame seeds

Arroz con Pollo: 1 ½ cups cooked Spanish-style rice with 4 oz. chicken and ¼ cup peas, served with 1 slice fresh bread and 1 tsp. butter or margarine

Linguine with White Clam Sauce: 1 ½ cups cooked linguine and approximately ⅔ cup clam sauce, accompanied by 2 slices crusty bread, ½ cup Italian green beans, and 1 tsp. butter or margarine

Roasted Chicken Breast: 4 oz. breast of chicken (remove skin after cooking), served with 1 ½ cups mashed potatoes (prepared with 2 tsp. margarine or butter and 1 Tb. skim milk) and ½ cup steamed fresh broccoli

Pizza: 1 ½ slices (4 × 4 in. square) Sicilian deep-dish pizza with 1 topping (blot all the oil!), served with a small garden salad and 1 Tb. low-fat dressing

Asian Chicken Breast: 4 oz. grilled skinless chicken breast lightly brushed during cooking with hoisin sauce (available in Asian markets), served with 2 cups cooked thin noodles and ½ cup mixed Oriental-style vegetables topped with 6 chopped cashews

Baked Lasagna: 4-in. square lasagna (prepared with low-fat ricotta and mozzarella cheeses and lean ground beef), served with ½ cup steamed spinach and 2 slices crusty bread

AND
1 cup skim milk

CAN-DO **Snacks**

The Product Guide contains an extensive listing of approved snacks from which to choose. Be sure to refer to the Guide for portion sizes.

AFTERNOON SNACK
This is an important snack as most kids are very hungry after school. There's a long stretch from lunch until dinner, and kids will be eager for this one.

CHOOSE TWO ITEMS FROM THE SNACKS SECTION OF THE PRODUCT GUIDE, SUCH AS:

Pop Secret Popcorn Bar, Chocolate Flavor topping and a Dole fruit juice bar
Munch'ems Chili Cheese crackers and Pretzel Rods
Teddy Grahams, Vanilla, and chocolate crunch rice cakes

SELECT ONE

1 small apple	½ banana
1 small orange	1 cup cantaloupe or honeydew cubes
1 small nectarine	1¼ cups watermelon cubes
1 medium peach	1¼ cups whole strawberries
2 tangerines	12 fresh, sweet cherries
1 small pear	17 small grapes
2 plums	1 mini-box of raisins

AND

1 cup skim milk

EVENING SNACK

Lots of kids like to have something to "finish off" the meal. So the evening snack can be eaten right after dinner as dessert or later in the evening.

CHOOSE TWO ITEMS FROM THE SNACKS SECTION OF THE PRODUCT GUIDE, SUCH AS:

Nacho Cheese Tortilla Thins and Strawberry Splash Gushers fruit snack
½ oz. bag of Butter Popcorn and Starburst Blueberry Lemonade Fruit Juice Bar
chocolate Chunk Chewy Low Fat Granola Bar and Snackwell's cheese crackers

SELECT ONE

1 small apple	½ banana
1 small orange	1 cup cantaloupe or honeydew cubes
1 small nectarine	1¼ cups watermelon cubes
1 medium peach	1¼ cups whole strawberries
2 tangerines	12 fresh, sweet cherries
1 small pear	17 small grapes
2 plums	1 mini-box of raisins

2500

About the Product Guide

Last night in the grocery store, my kids asked for snacks. They had in mind Rice Krispie Treats, which are now available premade at about 90 calories apiece. Right next to them were Oreo granola bars, Chips Ahoy! granola bars, and m&m Kudos bars. What's a confused parent to do? There are so many individually packaged snack items to choose from these days that it's difficult to decide which is best. New products are appearing all the time. How can you tell which ones fit in with your child's calorie-level plan? Use the Product Guide that begins on page 115.

This guide lists more than 400 snacks and other foods that are on the "approved" list for the Can-Do Eating Plan. In the Product Guide, you will discover which snacks and other foods fall within Plan guidelines. If it's on my list, it's an acceptable snack.

You may notice that I list some Weight Watchers and Slim-Fast brand items. I've included them because they meet my calorie criteria. But if your child is uncomfortable about taking a "diet" item to school for lunch or a snack—fearing the kids will tease him—by all means make another choice.

With so many new products entering the market, it seems impossible to keep track of every acceptable choice. This list is as up-to-date and comprehensive as I could make it—the result of hours of trekking through the supermarket aisles in search of options. Feel free to add to the Product Guide any snacks you find which meet the snack guideline: **110 calories or less.**

As for packaging individual portions yourself at home—I would caution you that it is more of a temptation for your child, who knows that the "big" box of cookies is up there in the cabinet. I realize the prepackaged versions can be more expensive, but I think it's money well-spent.

To help you find your way around, the Product Guide is organized alphabetically into major food categories:

Cereals
Lunch Meats
Snacks
Soups

Snacks is the largest section and is broken down into smaller categories:

Cakes
Chips
Cookies
Crackers
Frozen desserts
Fruit (canned)
Fruit snacks
Popcorn/Nuts
Pretzels
Pudding/Gelatin
Rice cakes/Popcorn cakes
Snack bars

THE PRODUCT GUIDE

CEREALS

Cheerios	General Mills	I cup	110
Honey Nut Cheerios	General Mills	I cup	120
Multi-grain Cheerios	General Mills	I cup	110
Froot Loops	General Mills	I cup	120
Confetti Froot Loops	General Mills	I cup	120
Lucky Charms	General Mills	I cup	120
Wheaties	General Mills	I cup	110
Instant Oatmeal, apple cinnamon	H-O	I pack	130
Instant Oatmeal, regular	H-O	I pack	110
Instant Oatmeal, sweet & mellow	H-O	I pack	150
Corn Flakes	Kellogg's	I cup	110
Corn Pops	Kellegg's	I cup	110
Rice Krispies	Kellogg's	I ¼ cups	110
Rice Krispies Kaleido	Kellogg's	I ¼ cups	110
Apple Jacks	Kellogg's	I cup	110
Crispix	Kellogg's	I cup	110
Instant Cream of Wheat, apple cinnamon	Nabisco	I pack	130
Instant Cream of Wheat, burstin berry	Nabisco	I pack	130
Instant Cream of Wheat, peachy peach	Nabisco	I pack	130
Instant Cream of Wheat, smashin strawberry	Nabisco	I pack	130
Instant Cream of Wheat, original	Nabisco	I pack	100
Instant Cream of Wheat, brown sugar cinnamon	Nabisco	I pack	130
Instant Cream of Wheat, maple brown sugar	Nabisco	I pack	140
Trix	Post	I cup	120
Kix	Post	I ⅓ cups	120
Honey Comb	Post	I ⅓ cups	110

Product Name	Manufacturer	Portion Size	Calories
CEREALS (cont'd)			
Cocoa Puffs	Post	I cup	120
Alpha-bits with marsh-mallows	Post	I cup	120
Instant Oatmeal, regular flavor	Quaker	I pack	150
Instant Oatmeal, peaches & cream	Quaker	I pack	130
Instant Oatmeal, apples & cinnamon	Quaker	I pack	130
Kids Choice Oatmeal, strawberries 'n stuff	Quaker	I pack	140
Kids Choice Oatmeal, cinnamon graham cookie	Quaker	I pack	140
Kids Choice Oatmeal, radical raspberry	Quaker	I pack	150
Kids Choice Oatmeal, maple & brown sugar	Quaker	I pack	140
LUNCH MEATS			
Smoked Chicken Breast	Butterball	6 slices	60
Smoked White Turkey	Butterball	3 slices	70
Turkey Ham	Butterball	3 slices	70
Turkey Bologna	Butterball	3 slices	150
Turkey Salami	Butterball	3 slices	100
Light Bologna	Deli Select (Hillshire Farms)	6 slices	80
Smoked Chicken Breast	Deli Select (Hillshire Farms)	6 slices	50
Smoked Turkey Breast	Deli Select (Hillshire Farms)	6 slices	60
Oven Roasted Chicken Breast	Deli Select (Hillshire Farms)	6 slices	50
Honey Ham	Deli Select (Hillshire Farms)	6 slices	60
Turkey Ham	Healthy Choice	6 slices	60
Oven-Roasted Turkey Breast	Healthy Favorites (Oscar Mayer)	4 slices	40
Smoked Cooked Ham	Healthy Favorites (Oscar Mayer)	4 slices	50

Product Name	Manufacturer	Portion Size	Calories
LUNCH MEATS (cont'd)			
Baked Ham	Healthy Favorites (Oscar Mayer)	4 slices	50
Oven Roasted Chicken Breast	Weaver Premium	3 slices	90
Oven Roasted Turkey Breast	Weaver Premium	3 slices	90
White Meat Chicken Roll	Weaver Premium	3 slices	90
SNACKS:			
Cakes			
Sweet Rewards, brownie	Betty Crocker (General Mills)	I bar	90
Sweet Rewards, double fudge supreme brownie	Betty Crocker (General Mills)	I bar	110
Cinnamon Crumb Coffee Cake	Hostess	I individual cake	80
Chocolate Frosted Brownie	Weight Watchers	I brownie	100
Chips			
Yellow Corn Chips	Arrowhead Mills	¾ oz.	90
Yellow Corn Chips with Cheese	Arrowhead Mills	¾ oz.	90
Lite Cheddar Puffs	Bearito	I cup	75
Cheeze Doodles	Borden	I bag (21 grams) ¾ oz.	110
Potato Chips	Cape Cod	⅝ oz. bag	90
Smart Temptation Tortilla Chips	Charlotte Charles Inc.	I oz.	100
Ripples Potato Chips	Eagle Snacks	I bag (½ oz.)	80
Cheese Crunch	Eagle Snacks	I bag (⅝ oz.)	100
Thins Potato Chips	Eagle Snacks	I bag (½ oz.)	80
Pretzel Mini-Bites	Eagle Snacks	I bag (9/16 oz.)	60

Product Name	Manufacturer	Portion Size	Calories
SNACKS (cont'd)			
Nacho Cheese Tortilla Thins	Eagle Snacks	1 bag (9/16 oz.)	80
Ruffles Potato Chips	Frito-Lay	1 package (½ oz.)	80
Doritos cheesier nacho	Frito-Lay	1 package (9/16 oz.)	80
Fritos Corn Chips	Frito-Lay	¾ oz. (24 chips)	120
Chee-tos Cheese Flavored Snacks—paws	Frito-Lay	1 package (⅝ oz.)	100
Lay's Potato Chips	Frito Lay	½ oz. (14 grams)	80
Baked Lay's Original Potato Crisps	Frito-Lay	1 oz. (about 12 chips)	110
Chee-tos Cheese Flavored Snacks—crunchy	Frito-Lay	1 package, (⅝ oz.)	100
Baked Lays	Frito-Lay	1 oz. (12 chips)	110
Baked Tortilla Chips	Guiltless Gourmet	1 oz. (12 chips)	110
Baked Tortilla Chips, nacho	Guiltless Gourmet	1 oz. (20 chips)	110
No Oil Corn Chips	Happy Heart	⅜ oz.	40
No Oil Corn Chips, cheddar	Happy Heart	⅜ oz.	40
No Oil Corn Chips, B-B-Q	Happy Heart	⅜ oz.	40
No Oil Corn Chips, nacho cheese	Happy Heart	⅜ oz.	40
Cheddar Lites	Healthy Valley	½ oz.	80
Mr. Phipps Tater Crisps, original	Nabisco	½ oz. (11 crisps)	60
Mr. Phipps Tater Crisps, ranch	Nabisco	½ oz. (11 crisps)	60

Product Name	Manufacturer	Portion Size	Calories
SNACKS (cont'd)			
Mr. Phipps Tater Crisps, sour cream & onion	Nabisco	½ oz. (11 crisps)	60
Smart Doodles with Cheese	Robert's American Gourmet	1 oz.	68
Smart Puffs with Real Wisconsin Cheese	Robert's American Gourmet	1 ¾ cups	110
Cheese Curls	Slim Fast	1 oz.	110
Light 'n Tasty Cheese Curls	Ultra Slim Fast	1 bag (1 oz.)	110
Corn Snackers	Weight Watchers	½ oz.	60
Potato Snacks, cheddar cheese	Weight Watchers	½ oz.	60
Potato Snacks, B-B-Q	Weight Watchers	½ oz.	60
Cookies			
Gingersnap	Archway	4 cookies	100
Oatmeal Chocolate Chip	Entenmann	2 cookies	80
Raisin Oatmeal	Health Valley	4 cookies	100
Chocolate Flavor Chip	Health Valley Health Chips	3 cookies	100
Teddy Grahams, Rockin Bears	Nabisco	11 cookies	60
Teddy Grahams, chocolate	Nabisco	11 cookies	60
Teddy Grahams, vanilla	Nabisco	11 cookies	60
Teddy Grahams, cinnamon	Nabisco	11 cookies	60
Dizzy Grizzlies Frosted Grahams with Sprinkles	Nabisco	5 cookies	93
SnackWell's Cinnamon Graham	Nabisco	9 pieces	50
SnackWell's Chocolate Chip	Nabisco	10 pieces	100

Product Name	Manufacturer	Portion Size	Calories
SNACKS (cont'd)			
Low-Fat Honey Maid Graham Crackers, cinnamon	Nabisco	2 full sheets	110
Low-Fat Honey Maid Graham Crackers, honey	Nabisco	2 full sheets	110
Nilla Wafers	Nabisco	3 wafers	60
Lorna Doone Shortbread	Nabisco	3 cookies	105
Chocolate Chip	Pepperidge Farm	1 pouch	100
Sugar Cookies	Pepperidge Farm	1 pouch	100
Ginger Man	Pepperidge Farm	1 pouch	70
Sugar Wafers	Sunshine	2 cookies	90
Lemon Coolers	Sunshine	3 cookies	90
Oatmeal Spice	Weight Watchers	1 package (3 cookies)	80
Shortbread Cookies	Weight Watchers	1 package (3 cookies)	80
Chocolate Chip	Weight Watchers	1 package (2 cookies)	90
Crackers			
Spud Baked Potato Snacks	Auburn Farms	25 crisps (1 oz.)	110
Munch'ems, original	Keebler	14 crackers	60
Munch'ems, nacho	Keebler	14 crackers	60
Munch'ems, cheddar	Keebler	13 crackers	60
Munch'ems, chili cheese	Keebler	13 crackers	60
Munch'ems, sour cream & onion	Keebler	13 crackers	60
Munch'ems, ranch	Keebler	14 crackers	90
Snorkels, pizza	Nabisco	27 crackers	70
Snorkels, cheddar	Nabisco	27 crackers	70
Snorkels, ranch	Nabisco	27 crackers	70

Product Name	Manufacturer	Portion Size	Calories
SNACKS (cont'd)			
Zings, original	Nabisco	15 crackers	70
Zings, cheddar	Nabisco	15 crackers	70
Zings, ranch	Nabisco	15 crackers	70
Ritz Ark Animals	Nabisco	35 crackers	100
Ritz Bits, cheese	Nabisco	6 sandwiches	80
Ritz Bits, cheese pizza	Nabisco	5 sandwiches	80
Ritz Bits, peanut butter	Nabisco	6 sandwiches	70
Ritz Bits, nacho cheese	Nabisco	6 sandwiches	80
Premium Bits	Nabisco	16 bits (½ oz.)	70
Wheat Thins Air Crisps	Nabisco	20 pieces	110
Ritz Air Crisps	Nabisco	18 crackers	110
No Fries, Tortilla Snack Crackers, salsa & sour cream	Pacific Grain	30 pieces (30 grams)	110
Goldfish, original	Pepperidge Farm	½ oz.	60
Goldfish, pretzel	Pepperidge Farm	43 pieces	110
Goldfish, cheddar	Pepperidge Farm	42 pieces	110
Frozen Desserts			
Healthy Temptations Snack Sandwiches	Betty Crocker	1 Sandwich	80
Fruit 'N Yogurt Bars, strawberry	Dole	1 bar	70
Fruit 'N Yogurt Bars, strawberry-banana	Dole	1 bar	70
Fruit 'N Yogurt Bars, mixed berry	Dole	1 bar	70
Fruit 'N Yogurt Bars, cherry	Dole	1 bar	80
Fruit 'N Cream, raspberry	Dole	1 bar	80

Product Name	Manufacturer	Portion Size	Calories
SNACKS (cont'd)			
Fruit 'N Cream, straw-berry	Dole	I bar	80
Sun Tops, punch	Dole	I bar	40
Sun Tops, lemonade	Dole	I bar	40
Sun Tops, grape	Dole	I bar	40
Sun Tops, orange	Dole	I bar	40
Yogurt Bars, chocolate	Dole	I bar	70
Fruit Lites, cherry	Dole	I bar	25
Fruit Lites, lemon	Dole	I bar	25
Fruit Lites, raspberry	Dole	I bar	25
Fruit Lites, pineapple-orange	Dole	I bar	25
Fruit 'n Juice, dark cherry	Dole	I bar	70
Fruit 'n Juice, peach pas-sion	Dole	I bar	70
Fruit 'n Juice, pineapple	Dole	I bar	70
Fruit 'n Juice, pine-orange	Dole	I bar	70
Fruit 'n Juice, raspberry	Dole	I bar	70
Fruit 'n Juice, strawberry	Dole	I bar	70
Juice Pops, all flavors	Dole	I bar	45
7-Up Spot Pops	DCA Food Ind.	I pop	30
Popsicle Juice Jets	Good Humor	I bar	45
Popsicle Ice Pops, all fla-vors	Good Humor	I pop	45
Lick-a-Color Popsicles, all flavors	Good Humor	I bar	50
Creamsicle	Good Humor	I bar	110
Fudgsicle, fudge pop	Good Humor	I bar	60
Fudgsicle, vanilla pop	Good Humor	I bar	60
Fudgsicle, chocolate-vanilla swirl	Good Humor	I bar	60
Minute Maid Fruit Juice Flavored Juice Ice Bar	Good Humor	I bar	60
Sorbet, wild berry	Häagen-Dazs	I bar	90

Product Name	Manufacturer	Portion Size	Calories
SNACKS (cont'd)			
Sorbet, chocolate	Häagen-Dazs	1 bar	80
Frozen Yogurt Fruit Bars, all flavors	Häagen-Dazs	1 bar	70
Colombo Chocolate Sorbet	Integrated Brands, Inc	1 bar	60
Fla-Vor-Ice	The Jel Sert Company	1 pop	30
Pop-Ice	The Jel Sert Company	1 bar	20
Gelatin Pops, Raspberry, Orange	Jell-O	1 pop	35
Snowburst Bars, lemon	Jell-O	1 bar	45
Snowburst Bars, orange	Jell-O	1 bar	45
Lite Sandwich	Klondike	1 sandwich	90
Kool Pops, all Flavors	Kool-Aid	1 pop	40
Kool-Aid Pumps	Kool-Aid	1 pop	80
Flavor Pops	Life Saver	1 bar	40
Natural Fruit Juice Bars	Lucerne	1 bar	85
Twin Pops	Lucerne	1 pop	60
Mini Pops	Lucerne	1 pop	40
Starburst Fruit Juice Bars, Lemonade Blends, all flavors	m & m Mars	1 bar	50
Starburst Low-fat Frozen Yogurt Cups, fruit blends	m & m Mars	1 cup	90
Flintstone Push-up Pop, cherry	Nestlé	1 pop	90
Flintstone Push-up Pop, grape	Nestlé	1 pop	90
Flintstone Push-up Pop, orange	Nestlé	1 pop	90
Flintstone Push-up Pop, lime	Nestlé	1 pop	90
Flintstone Push-up Pop berry	Nestlé	1 pop	90

Product Name	Manufacturer	Portion Size	Calories
SNACKS (cont'd)			
Flintstone Push-up Sherbet Treats, all flavors	Nestlé	1 tube	100
Quik Milk Chocolate Ice Cream Pop	Nestlé	1 pop	80
Funwiches	Nestlé	1 sandwich	110
Exploding Pops	Nestlé	1 pop	70
Big Stick Ice Pops, orange	Popsicle	1 pop	80
Firecracker Ice Pop	Popsicle	1 pop	40
Ice Pops	Popsicle	1 pop	50
Trix Pop, all flavors	Steve's Homemade Ice Cream	1 pop	40
Trix Pop, Fudge n' Fruity	Steve's Homemade Ice Cream	1 pop	80
Yoo Hoo Fudge Bars	Steve's Homemade Ice Cream	1 bar	70
Great American Chilly Pops	Steve's Homemade Ice Cream	1 bar	40
Chocolate Treat	Weight Watchers	1 bar	100
Fruit Juice Bars, all flavors	Welch's	1.75 oz. bar	45
Fruit Juice Bars, all flavors	Welch's	3 oz. bar	80
Fruit (canned)			
Fruit Naturals, Pineapple Tidbits (no sugar added)	Del Monte	4.5 oz.	90
Mixed Fruit, Heavy Syrup	Del Monte	4.5 oz.	100
Diced Pears, Extra Light Syrup	Del Monte	4.5 oz.	60
Diced Peaches, Heavy Syrup	Del Monte	4.5 oz.	90
Diced Peaches, Extra Light Syrup	Del Monte	4.5 oz.	60
Natural Lite Mixed Fruit	Libby's	4.5 oz.	60
Natural Lite Yellow Cling Diced Peaches	Libby's	4.5 oz.	50

Product Name	Manufacturer	Portion Size	Calories
SNACKS (cont'd)			
Applesauce & Strawberries	Mott's	3.9 oz.	80
Applesauce & Mixed Fruit	Mott's	3.9 oz.	80
Applesauce, Natural Style (unsweetened)	Mott's	4 oz.	50
Applesauce, original flavor	Mott's	4 oz.	50
Fruit Snacks			
String Thing, cherry	Betty Crocker (General Mills)	1 pouch	80
String Thing, berry	Betty Crocker (General Mills)	1 pouch	80
Fruit Snackers, beasty bites	Brook Candy Co.	1 pouch	90
Fruit Snackers, Pinocchio	Brook Candy Co.	1 pouch	90
Fruit Snackers, little monsters	Brook Candy Co.	1 pouch	100
Fruit Snackers, Peter Pan	Brook Candy Co.	1 pouch	90
Creepy Crawlers	Farley's	1 pouch	90
Basket Buddies	Farley's	1 pouch	90
Michael Jordan	Farley's	1 pouch	90
Zoo Animals	Farley's	1 pouch	90
Dinosaurs	Farley's	1 pouch	90
Teenage Mutant Ninja Turtles	Farley's	1 pouch	90
Cowboys of Moomesa	Farley's	1 pouch	90
Trolls	Farley's	1 pouch	90
Trolls in Trouble, cherry	Farley's	1 pouch	80
Scary	Farley's	1 pouch	90
Cherry	Farley's	1 pouch	90
Grape	Farley's	1 pouch	90
Strawberry	Farley's	1 pouch	90
Zoo Animals	Farley's	1 pouch	90
Flintstone Real Fruit Snacks	Ferrara Pan	1 pouch	100

Product Name	Manufacturer	Portion Size	Calories
SNACKS (cont'd)			
Fruit Roll-up, grape	General Mills	1 roll	50
Fruit Roll-up, strawberry	General Mills	1 roll	50
Fruit Roll-up, cherry	General Mills	1 roll	50
Fruit Roll-up, Hot Colors, blastin berry	General Mills	1 roll	55
Fruit Roll-up, Crazy Colors, berry banana	General Mills	1 roll	55
Fruit Roll-up, Peel 'n Build	General Mills	1 roll	55
Fruit by the Foot, grape	General Mills	1 roll	80
Fruit by the Foot, strawberry	General Mills	1 roll	80
Fruit by the Foot, rainbow punch	General Mills	1 roll	80
Fruit by the Foot, cherry	General Mills	1 roll	80
Fruit by the Foot, color by the foot	General Mills	1 roll	80
Soda Licious	General Mills	1 pouch	100
Gushers, strawberry splash	General Mills	1 pouch	90
Gushers, wild cherry	General Mills	1 pouch	90
Gushers, gushin grape	General Mills	1 pouch	90
Gushers, fruitomic punch	General Mills	1 pouch	90
Shark Bites, fruit punch	General Mills	1 pouch	100
Shark Bites, assorted fruit	General Mills	1 pouch	100
Rollerblade	General Mills	1 pouch	90
Berry Bears, fruit punch	General Mills	1 pouch	100
Berry Bears, assorted fruit	General Mills	1 pouch	100
Surf's Up!	General Mills	1 pouch	100
Tasmanian Devil	General Mills	1 pouch	90
Bugs Bunny	General Mills	1 pouch	90
The Jetsons	Lipton	1 pouch	100
Real Fruit Bars, raspberry	Nature's Choice	1 bar	50
Wacky Players, football	Sunkist	1 pouch	100

Product Name	Manufacturer	Portion Size	Calories
SNACKS (cont'd)			
Wacky Players, basketball	Sunkist	1 pouch	100
California Sundried Raisins, mini box	Sunmaid	1 box (14.1 grams)	45
Fruit Snack, cinnamon	Weight Watchers	½ oz.	50
Apple Chips	Weight Watchers	¾ oz.	70
Popcorn / Nuts			
Jolly Time, natural light microwave popcorn	American Pop Corn Company	3 cups	72
Pop Secret—By Request, natural and butter microwave popcorn	Betty Crocker (General Mills)	3 cups	65
Pop Secret Lite Butter microwave popcorn	Betty Crocker (General Mills)	3 cups	70
Original Lite Popcorn	Boston Popcorn Company	½ oz. bag	60
Butter Toffee Glazed Popcorn	Cracker Jack (Borden)	1 cup	110
Smart Pop microwave popcorn	Orville Redenbacher	3 cups	40
Natural Light Microwave Popcorn	Orville Redenbacher	3 cups	60
Popcorn, lightly buttered	Smart Food	½ oz.	70
Popcorn with white cheddar cheese	Smart Food	1 package	100
Smart Snackers Honey Roasted Peanuts	Weight Watchers	1 pouch	100
Smart Snackers Caramel Popcorn	Weight Watchers	1 pack	199
Butter Popcorn	Wise (Borden)	1 bag (½ oz.)	80
Pretzels			
Pretzel Stix	Bachman	1 oz. box	110
Pretzel Mini-Bites	Eagle Snacks	1 bag (9/16 oz.)	60

Product Name	Manufacturer	Portion Size	Calories
SNACKS (cont'd)			
Handi snack, Cheese'n pretzels	Kraft	1 pack (1.1 oz.)	110
Mr. Phipps Pretzel Chips, Original	Nabisco	8 pretzel chips	60
Mr. Phipps Pretzel Chips, Lite salt	Nabisco	8 pretzel chips	60
Mr. Phipps Pretzel Chips, Cinnamon	Nabisco	8 pretzel chips	60
Mini Pretzel Twists	Quinlan (Borden)	1 bag (28 grams)	110
Pretzel Twists	Rold Gold	1 oz. (10 twists)	110
Pretzel Rods	Rold Gold	1 oz. (3 rods)	110
Pretzel Sticks	Rold Gold	1 oz. (50 sticks)	110
Pretzel, Tiny Twists	Rold Gold	1 oz. (15 tiny twists)	110
Pretzel Twists	Ultra Slim Fast	1 oz. bag	100
Pudding / Gelatin			
Light Snack Cup, vanilla	Del Monte	4.25 oz.	100
Light Snack Cup, chocolate	Del Monte	4.25 oz.	100
Chocolate Pudding Free	Hershey	4 oz.	100
Snack Pack Lite Pudding, chocolate	Hunt's	4 oz.	100
Snack Pack Lite Pudding, tapioca	Hunt's	4 oz.	100
Light Pudding Snack, chocolate	Jell-O	4 oz.	100
Light Pudding Snack, chocolate fudge	Jell-O	4 oz.	100
Light Pudding Snack, vanilla	Jell-O	4 oz.	100

Product Name	Manufacturer	Portion Size	Calories
SNACKS (cont'd)			
Light Pudding Snack, chocolate/vanilla	Jell-O	4 oz.	100
Gelatin, orange	Jell-O	3.5 oz.	80
Gelatin, strawberry	Jell-O	3.5 oz.	80
Gelatin, banana	Jell-O	3.5 oz.	80
Gelatin, cherry	Jell-O	3.5 oz.	80
Gelatin, raspberry	Jell-O	3.5 oz.	80
Butterscotch Pudding	Slim-Fast	4 oz.	100
Chocolate Pudding	Slim-Fast	4 oz.	100
Vanilla Pudding	Slim-Fast	4 oz.	100
Chocolate Pudding Lite	Swiss Miss	4 oz.	100
Rice Cakes / Popcorn Cakes			
Rice Snax, original	Amsnack, Inc.	½ oz.	60
Rice Snax, chili cheddar	Amsnack, Inc.	½ oz.	60
Popcorn Cakes, butter	Chico San	1 cake	40
Rice Cakes, cinnamon crunch	Chico San	1 cake	60
Popcorn Cakes, white cheddar	Chico San	1 cake	50
Popcorn Cakes, caramel	Chico San	1 cake	50
Butter Popcorn Cakes	Gifts of Nature	5 cakes	70
Caramel Popcorn Cakes	Gifts of Nature	5 cakes	50
Mini Rice Cakes, honey nut	Hain Pure Food Company	½ oz.	60
Mini Rice Cakes, apple cinnamon	Hain Pure Food Company	½ oz.	60
Mini Rice Cakes, plain	Hain Pure Food Company	½ oz. (6 cakes)	60
Mini Rice Cakes, teriyaki	Hain Pure Food Company	½ oz. (5 cakes)	50
Mini Rice Cakes, nacho cheese	Hain Pure Food Company	½ oz.	70
Mini Rice Cakes, cheese	Hain Pure Food Company	5 cakes	60

Product Name	Manufacturer	Portion Size	Calories
SNACKS (cont'd)			
Mini Popcorn Cakes	Hain Pure Food Company	½ oz.	60
Corn Rice Cakes	Nature Food	1 cake	45
Buckwheat Cakes	Nature Food	1 cake	45
Mini Crispys, honey almond	Pacific Rice Products	1 cake	12
Mini Crispys, apple spice	Pacific Rice Products	2 cakes	30
Mini Crispys, teriyaki	Pacific Rice Products	1 cake	12
Rice Snax, Santa Fe cheddar	Pacific Lites	1 ¾ cups (1 oz.)	100
Rice Cakes, regular	Quaker	1 cake	35
Rice Cakes, apple cinnamon	Quaker	1 cake	50
Rice Cakes, cinnamon crunch	Quaker	1 cake	50
Rice Cakes, chocolate crunch	Quaker	1 cake	50
Popcorn Cakes, blueberry crunch	Quaker	1 cake	50
Popcorn Cakes, strawberry crunch	Quaker	1 cake	50
Rice Cakes, banana nut	Quaker	1 cake	50
Popcorn Cakes, caramel	Quaker	1 cake	50
Popcorn Cakes, regular	Quaker	1 cake	35
Popcorn Cakes, nacho	Quaker	1 cake	40
Popcorn Cakes, butter	Quaker	1 cake	35
Popcorn Cakes, white cheddar	Quaker	1 cake	40
Wheat Cakes	Quaker	1 cake	40
Wheat Cakes, lightly salted	Quaker	1 cake	35
Mini Rice Cakes, apple cinnamon	Quaker	5 mini cakes (½ oz.)	50
Mini Rice Cakes, white cheddar	Quaker	6 mini cakes	50

Product Name	Manufacturer	Portion Size	Calories
SNACKS (cont'd)			
Mini Rice Cakes, caramel corn	Quaker	5 mini cakes	50
Mini Rice Cakes, chocolate crunch	Quaker	5 mini cakes	50
Mini Rice Cakes, honey nut	Quaker	5 mini cakes	50
Popcorn Cakes, white cheddar	Spiral	1 cake	50
Snack Bars			
Pop-Secret Popcorn Bars, caramel topping	Betty Crocker (General Mills)	1 bar	80
Pop-Secret Popcorn Bars, chocolate topping	Betty Crocker (General Mills)	1 bar	80
Marshmallow Munchie, original	Campfire	1 bar	100
Marshmallow Munchie, chocolate chip	Campfire	1 bar	110
Sweet Escapes, Chocolate Toffee Crisp Bars	Hershey's	1 bar	80
Sweet Escapes, Caramel & Peanut Butter Crispy Bars	Hershey's	1 bar	80
Sweet Escapes, Triple Chocolate Wafer Bars	Hershey's	1 bar	80
Low Fat Granola Bar, crunchy oats	Kellogg's	1 bar	80
Low Fat Granola Bar, almonds & brown sugar	Kellogg's	1 bar	80
Low Fat Granola Bar, apple spice	Kellogg's	1 bar	80
Low Fat Granola Bar, cinnamon raisin	Kellogg's	1 bar	80
Rice Krispies Treats	Kellogg's	1 bar	90

Product Name	Manufacturer	Portion Size	Calories
SNACKS (cont'd)			
Dream Bar (caramel and nougat in real milk chocolate)	Litesse	1 bar	90
Kudos, chocolate chunk	m&m Mars	1 bar	90
Kudos, honey nut	m&m Mars	1 bar	90
Kudos, Dove chocolate chunk	m&m Mars	1 bar	90
Kudos, m&m	m&m Mars	1 bar	90
SnackWell's Fudge Dipped Granola Bar, original	Nabisco	1 bar	110
SnackWell's Fudge Dipped Granola Bar, oatmeal raisin	Nabisco	1 bar	110
SnackWell's Fudge Dipped Granola Bar, caramel	Nabisco	1 bar	110
Low Fat Chewy Granola Bar, chocolate chip	Nature Valley	1 bar	110
Low Fat Chewy Granola Bar, oatmeal raisin	Nature Valley	1 bar	110
Low Fat Chewy Granola Bar, honey nut	Nature Valley	1 bar	110
Low Fat Chewy Granola Bar, apple brown sugar	Nature Valley	1 bar	110
Raspberry Filled Cereal Bars	Nature's Choice	1 bar	110
Chewy Low Fat Granola Bars, chocolate chunk	Quaker	1 bar	110
Chewy Low Fat Granola Bars, apple berry	Quaker	1 bar	110
Chewy Low Fat Granola Bars, s'mores	Quaker	1 bar	110

Product Name	Manufacturer	Portion Size	Calories
SNACKS (cont'd)			
Chewy Low Fat Granola Bars, cookies 'n cream	Quaker	1 bar	110
Chewy Low Fat Granola Bars, oatmeal cookie	Quaker	1 bar	110
Low Fat Chewy Granola Bar, chocolate mint	Quaker	1 bar	110
SOUPS			
Chicken Flavor Vegetable Soup	Knorr	1 envelope	100
Chicken Vegetable	Lipton Cup-A-Soup	1 envelope	50
Hearty Chicken	Lipton Cup-A-Soup	1 envelope	60
Spring Vegetable	Lipton Cup-A-Soup	1 envelope	50
Ring Noodle, Chicken Flavor	Lipton Cup-A-Soup	1 envelope	50
Chicken Noodle	Lipton Cup-A-Soup	1 envelope	50
Cream of Chicken	Lipton Cup-A-Soup	1 envelope	70
Chicken Supreme	Lipton Cup-A-Soup	1 envelope	90
Green Pea	Lipton Cup-A-Soup	1 envelope	100
Cream of Mushroom	Lipton Cup-A-Soup	1 envelope	60
Tomato	Lipton Cup-A-Soup	1 envelope	90
Chicken Flavor	Nissin Mug Noodles	0.8 oz.	100
Beef Flavor	Nissin Mug Noodles	0.8 oz.	100
Oriental Flavor	Nissin Mug Noodles	0.8 oz.	100
Beef Minestrone	Progresso	1 cup	140
Beef Noodle	Progresso	1 cup	140
Beef Barley	Progresso	1 cup	130
Chicken Barley	Progresso	1 cup	110
Chicken & Wild Rice	Progresso	1 cup	100
Chicarina Chicken Soup with Meatballs	Progresso	1 cup	120
Chicken Rice with vegetables	Progresso	1 cup	110

Product Name	Manufacturer	Portion Size	Calories
SOUPS (cont'd)			
Homestyle Chicken with vegetables and maca-roni pearls	Progresso	1 cup	100
Chicken minestrone	Progresso	1 cup	120
Hearty Penne in chicken broth	Progresso	1 cup	70
Minestrone, original recipe	Progresso	1 cup	130
Hearty Minestrone and shells	Progresso	1 cup	120
Broccoli and Shells in Chicken Broth	Progresso	1 cup	70
Beef Vegetable and Rotini	Progresso	1 cup	120
Meatballs and Pasta Pearls in Chicken Broth	Progresso	1 cup	140
Lentils and Shells	Progresso	1 cup	130
Hearty Tomato and Ro-tini	Progresso	1 cup	90
Hearty Vegetable and Rotini	Progresso	1 cup	110
Tomato Tortellini	Progresso	1 cup	120
Tomato	Progresso	1 cup	90
Vegetable	Progresso	1 cup	90
Lentil	Progresso	1 cup	140

7

The Final Ingredient:
How Physical Exercise Ensures Success

By now, it may seem as if I have shared with you everything I know about weight-management success. You've met with your child's doctor. You've seen the menus. You've paged through the Product Guide and stocked your pantry. But there is one more essential component to this plan, an ingredient that will ensure your child's weight-control success, now and for a lifetime. Exercise.

Remember, weight management is about balancing calories-in and calories-out. The body uses up calories-in by moving around, so the more moving around, the more calories-out. By adding regular exercise into the equation, you can forget about counting fat grams, forget about counting calories. Instead, think about movement. Play. Exercise!

There's nothing like exercise to change the calories-in, calories-out equation. More calories-out means more fat burned. For example, Heather, a young girl I've been working with, came in to see me recently. Stepping onto the scale with a guilty smile, she was surprised to learn she had lost some weight. She felt compelled to reveal her secret: She had been sneaking candy bars and hiding them from her mother quite successfully all summer long! Why, then, the weight loss? Since it was summertime, she was biking and swimming a lot—

changing the number of calories-out in a way that took care
of the increased calories-in. I let her know that if she kept up
her exercise level, she would be able to continue indulging in
the occasional treat. The simple input-output explanation
made sense to her, and she managed to keep up the good
work even after the weather turned colder that fall.

Exercise really helps.

Physical fitness advocate Arnold Schwarzenegger cites nu-
merous benefits to exercise in his book *Fitness for Kids*: "Exercise plays a key role in helping young people develop
important motor skills such as agility, coordination, and balance. They have better posture, they sleep and move better,
recover more quickly from sickness and injury, have more endurance and concentration, and can handle physical emergen-
cies more easily than unfit kids." What's more, kids who
regularly participate in sports or other physical activities build
self-esteem as they learn new skills, and they feel good about
socializing with their peers. These are just some of the benefits
exercise has to offer.

If you yourself don't like exercise and were hoping this plan
would be as simple as controlling calories-in, you're probably
not alone. Adults often hope their own "starvation" diets will
cause them to shed pounds quickly without the need for a
permanent lifestyle change. Despite an ongoing fitness craze

FAST FACT: Peanut Butter Blues

Unfortunately, reduced-fat peanut butter does not net a calorie
savings. Regular peanut butter has 16 grams of fat and 190 calories
per 2 Tb. serving. Reduced-fat peanut butter is almost the same: 12
to 13 grams of fat and the same 190 calories per serving.

Why? What the reduced-fat spreads lack in peanuts is made up
for with corn syrup or maltodextrin and soy bean protein. What
manufacturers take out in fat calories, they make up for with other
ingredients.

in this country, a lot of us still react with fear and trepidation when we hear the e-word.

But I cannot overemphasize the importance of exercise. I firmly believe that reducing caloric intake without adding exercise is a waste of time. And research backs me up. The fact is, the pounds may drop off at first with just a reduction in calories, but in time, the body responds to a decrease in calories by burning calories more slowly. This means that extra calories will be stored, and storing calories means weight gain—which is exactly what you wanted to avoid.

Physical activity is especially important for children with weight problems. Because children's bodies are steadily growing and changing, their caloric needs are great. Overly restricting their caloric intake jeopardizes growth and nutrition. The solution? Limiting caloric intake to the right amount per day, then adding exercise so those extra calories get burned up instead of stored.

Very simply, if you don't put exercise into the equation, then you have to reduce calories much more significantly. The problem is, it's harder to stay with a restrictive diet over the long haul, especially for kids. Adding exercise allows for a more liberal eating plan. The bonus: Very active kids don't have to think about what they are eating. They eat when they're hungry, they eat until they're full, and that's that. I tell my patients, "The more you move around, the more liberal we can be about the food choices you make." That makes sense to them.

Why It Works

Of the many benefits of exercise, there are three that stand out when it comes to weight management. First, physical activity burns calories. The more rigorous the activity, the more calories burned. Walking, for instance, is a good, steady calorie burner. But jogging or doing aerobic dance burns even more calories. Second, the body not only burns calories at a higher rate during exercise, but also continues to do so at a higher rate for a few hours afterward, extending the calorie-burning effect.

Finally, and perhaps most important, regular exercise actually changes the way the body uses calories, and that is what makes ongoing regular physical activity such an essential part of weight management. "Becoming fit can alter one's physiology," says Philip Walker of the Cooper Clinic in Dallas. A more fit body makes better use of the fuel it takes in. How? Exercise helps people to burn fat and gain muscle, so fit people have a higher proportion of muscle. And since muscle tissue requires more calories than fat-storing tissue, a fit person can eat more calories without gaining weight.

On the other hand, when you consume fewer calories without exercising regularly, the body's survival mechanism kicks in—it senses that there is less food available and so makes an adjustment. The body's metabolism slows down, fewer calories are burned, and the weight stays on.

Exercising more while controlling calorie intake is the complete solution to overweight. But beyond weight control, there are many other long-term health benefits to exercising regularly. For one, regular exercise reportedly strengthens the heart and lungs, decreases the risk of developing diabetes, osteoporosis, and some cancers, reduces stress, fights depression, and counteracts the effects of aging. Perhaps most important for your child is that she will *feel* better—move better, have more energy, make more friends, and have more fun—when she is more fit. Having something to do, whether it's shooting baskets in the driveway or going to soccer practice, also keeps kids busy and out of the kitchen.

What Is Exercise?

When you think of exercise, do you envision organized sports, strenuous workouts on complicated equipment—and arguments and resistance from your usually sedentary child? If your couch potato flatly refuses to play tennis, join the soccer team, or swim laps at the neighborhood pool after school, asking him to exercise may seem like asking for trouble. You know your child will refuse, so why bother?

But you don't have to force exercise. You don't have to beg your child to do it. You don't even have to call it exercise. All you need to do is find ways to get kids moving, and that's easier than you think. You can devise plenty of ways for your child to exercise without ever signing him up for tennis lessons or Little League. Emphasize fun. Downplay competition as much as possible, especially if an activity is new to your child.

Here are some popular physical activities that burn calories. Some are for little kids. Some are for big kids. Some are for kids of all ages. All of them are guaranteed to get your child moving.

Playing leapfrog with old pillows
Playing hide-and-seek outside
Playing hopscotch with sidewalk chalk
Going to The Discovery Zone or Leapin' Lizards
Climbing on monkey bars or a jungle gym
Running backyard relay races
Climbing a rope
Swinging on tire swing
Playing freeze tag
Rolling down a hill and running back up
Wrestling with parents, siblings, or friends
Maneuvering through a homemade obstacle course
Ice skating
Dancing to favorite music
Sledding (and carrying the sled back up the hill!)
Shoveling snow
Jumping rope alone or with friends
Pool activities: diving for pennies, Marco Polo, relay races
Backyard Slip 'n' Slide
Running through lawn sprinklers
In-line skating (Rollerblading)
Skateboarding

Catching fireflies
Playing driveway hockey
Playing balloon volleyball indoors
Playing Nerf basketball indoors
Throwing a Frisbee
Practicing soccer headers
Shooting hoops in the driveway or at the park
Tumbling on the family room carpet
Doing handstands and cartwheels outside
Walking—home from school, to the store, to a friend's
   house
Raking leaves
Hiking along a trail
Riding a bike around the block
Playing capture the flag
Playing Redlight-greenlight (start and stop)

The key is movement: Sustained physical movement that gets the pulse going a little faster and challenges the body. Skill is not always a prerequisite. When it comes to kids, the activity has to be fun and just a little bit breathtaking. If your child is breathing a little harder and starting to break into a sweat, then you know it's working.

Ten Modern Conveniences
That Keep Our Kids from Exercising

Remote-control television	Portable telephones
Automatic car washes	Multiple household telephone jacks
Household and yard help	Drive-through restaurants
Computers	Garage-door openers
Video games	Leaf blowers and snowblowers

When discussing the importance of physical activity with your child, let him know that it's an essential part of the Plan. Exercise and sensible eating go hand in hand. The more he exercises, the more food he will be able to burn off. Without exercise, your child would have to cut back too much on the foods he loves. Why be miserable and hungry when he can just get up and move around a little each day and still enjoy the foods he loves? Eating and exercise are a package deal. This is a new way of living, not a short-term "crash" diet, so it will work only if both the eating and the exercise components are in place.

Selecting an Activity

When I sit down with a patient to devise a fitness strategy, my method is always the same, whether the patient is male or female, younger or older. The suggestions I make are based on what I know about that child's particular interests and abilities—gender and age factor in, but they don't limit the possibilities. For instance, I might suggest that a girl put on some music and dance for half an hour, or that a boy go outside and shoot baskets, but I could just as easily reverse these suggestions if that seemed appropriate. To a younger child, I might suggest joining Mom for a walk with the dog or a family bike ride; I would assume a sixteen-year-old would prefer more independent activities.

To help my patients determine a fitness plan, I discuss the following questions with them and their parents:

1. Which activities do you enjoy most?
2. Which activities would you like to try?
3. Which of these activities will you be able to do regularly? Consider the following:
   a. *Convenience:* Suppose your son or daughter wants to take up ice hockey. Is the activity available in your area? Is it easy to get to? If not, he might be able to go skating only occasionally and would need to choose another activity as his main form of exercise.

b. *Cost:* Is the activity affordable? Horseback riding lessons may be your daughter's dream, but they probably aren't an everyday option, so a less expensive—or even free—activity would be a better staple.

c. *Seasonal nature:* If your child chooses swimming, will she be able to continue during the winter? If she chooses figure skating will she want to switch to an outdoor activity once the weather is nice? (An indoor pool will allow year-round swimming; Rollerblading can be a warm-weather skating alternative.)

d. *Effectiveness:* Some things look more like calorie burners than they really are. For example, bowling isn't the best choice for our purposes. If your child chooses a less active form of recreation, then supplement it with another, more active type of exercise.

How to Begin

You've talked with your health professional about your child's current fitness level, so you have some idea of where to start. If your child chooses to try a sport, it's a good idea to give him the chance to build up some strength, stamina, and skill before the pressure is really on to perform. If your child is overly challenged, his initial discouragement and frustration may kill his early enthusiasm for the activity. It's better to begin slowly, building up gradually. Keep in mind that your child has to contend not only with extra weight but also a possible lack of self-confidence after a long period of inactivity.

Sometimes, parents may be inclined to protect their child from engaging in certain activities because they don't see their child as an athlete. But most kids can ride a bike, go for a walk, or help in the garden. Remember, exercise is not just about team sports. It's about getting up and moving around. A child who is not a great soccer fullback still has some strength and can be fit and in condition. All children can find some area in which to develop fitness. To learn more about physical activities available in your area, contact the local parks and recreation department, the YMCA, or area day camps. Talk to other parents, too, to find out what their kids are interested in. When possible, sign your child up for activities with a friend. If you stay committed to physical activity as part of the program, your child will too. Provide the basics—comfortable clothing and athletic shoes, a few good ideas, the opportunity to invite friends to join in or sign up for a class together, a chance to brush up on some sports skills at home before taking a class or joining a team. Then let the fun begin.

Changes as They Age

Tailor your child's activities to age, ability, and interests. If she enjoys active play or sports, great. But everyone's different and if you force your child to do something she does not enjoy, it will only backfire. Seek your child's input and realize that she may try a few different activities before finding the one that is truly her thing. You may encounter some resistance to exercise, especially with an older child, who may feel embarrassed by a lack of athletic ability or even just the idea of wearing sports clothes such as shorts or a swimsuit. Whatever the activity, begin gradually, and be realistic. An overweight adolescent will not have success in an intermediate or advanced aerobics class. Being unable to keep up may cause your child to become frustrated enough to end an exercise program before it really begins. Younger kids, too, feel awkward, and may shy away from physical activities with others. Let them start one-on-one, taking walks with you, skating, or riding bikes. In time, the fitness bug will bite.

For Younger Children

Children up to age six or seven can usually get enough exercise in the form of unstructured play—running around the playground or in the backyard. Young kids naturally move around a lot, burning off calories, and they don't always need our help thinking of ways to do so. If they need ideas, turn to the list on pages 139–140 for suggestions. And if they have an interest in lessons, team sports, or other organized physical activities, so much the better. One caution: The American Academy of Pediatrics does not recommend structured infant exercise classes. Let your child's physical activity develop over time. He or she will express an interest in structured activities when the time is right.

For Older Children

By age eight or nine, organized sports start to become popular. As your child chooses an activity, keep in mind that some sports are more active than others. Soccer, swimming, lacrosse, and basketball are active. But softball can involve a lot more standing around, waiting for a hit ball or a turn at bat. Even if the softball coach has the team run around the field two or three times before practice, that's still not enough for a workout. Volleyball is another sport that may not offer much in the way of intense activity. If your child isn't sweaty and heated by the time it's over, you should supplement sports practice with other physical activities.

When older kids want to embark on a fitness program, encourage them to do so with a friend. As many adults know, having a workout buddy is a real motivator, and this is probably even more true for young people. With a fitness pal, your preteen or adolescent child will be more likely to stay with a class or program for a longer period of time. Even walking with a friend is more fun than walking alone, and you may feel your child is safer walking with someone else. And taking daily walks in preparation for an event such as a walk-a-thon is a great way to work toward a goal; just remember to keep up the same activity level after the walk-a-thon is over.

What Defines Physical Fitness?

You don't have to turn your child into an athlete. Physical fitness is about overall health, not skill at a particular sport. We hear about fitness a lot, perhaps most often from perfect-bodied exercise gurus on television. But don't let them scare you. Fitness is just good physical condition. There are several components to fitness:

- Healthy heart and lungs—to efficiently deliver oxygen to muscles, allowing them to perform their work.
- Muscle strength and endurance—the stronger the muscle, the more the body can move and the more endurance it has. Strong muscles and bones can hold back the aging process, and endurance means more energy for a longer period of time.
- Flexibility—the ability of joints and muscles to move smoothly and fully. Flexibility helps prevent injuries. Some people are naturally more flexible than others, but everyone can become more flexible through stretching and exercise.
- Body composition—the percentage of body fat versus the amount of lean muscle mass. Muscle tissue burns more calories than fat-storing tissue, so the more muscle you have the more calories you can eat.

Your child may be fit in some ways and not others. A child may be strong enough to hit a home run, but have trouble running around the bases because he has very little endurance. Or a child might naturally be very flexible even though he has very little lean muscle mass and a large percentage of body fat. Fitness is not about whether your child can hit a tennis ball or do a split. It's about total physical conditioning—fine-tuning the body machine. Everybody needs endurance, strength, and flexibility to be in good health.

Even so, fitness is not the first thing on your child's mind, even when that child has agreed to work on a weight problem. What do kids think about? From the hundreds of patients I've worked with, two reasons almost always surface as we talk about what motivates them: Kids want to do the things the other kids are doing, and they want to look better. They don't talk about a healthy heart and lungs. They don't talk about building muscles. They just want to feel good about themselves and be pretty much like everybody else. The remarkable thing is, regular fitness activities offer all this and more. Once your child has become physically fit, she will go forward in life as a team player who is willing to accept new challenges and practice hard to achieve mastery.

The Minimum

Your child should spend at least half an hour three times a week or more engaged in active play or continuous aerobic (heart-pumping) activity. That's what the American Academy of Pediatrics recommends in order for a child to be physically fit. For its calorie-burning value, more exercise is even better. If your child wants to exercise every day, that's terrific, especially when weight control is an issue. But never suggest that if your child can't exercise daily, he shouldn't do it at all.

It's okay to be sympathetic to your child's nervousness about being clumsy or out of shape, but don't accept repeated excuses. "Stomachaches" and "too much homework" are possible now and then, but "not enough time" doesn't cut it: Everyone has time for a half hour of exercise. I often remind my patients that I'm only talking about a "sitcom's worth" of time: Just half an hour. (A favorite half-hour television show makes a great exercise timer—just park a stationary bicycle in front of the screen and let your child go!)

Encourage your kids. Play with them. When they take an interest in sports or teams, explore your community's options and see what is available for them. But you need not force structured activities for young children. They don't need to jog around a track or swim laps. Active play is good enough so long as they remain interested in it. Kindergarten kids are excited these days about karate, and they kick and chop in the air all day long. Some parents might get tired of the accompanying cries of "Hi-yaaa!" but I'd suggest they think again: That much activity really does burn extra calories, and it promotes an interest in fitness and flexibility that will be a real plus as your child gets older. If the yelling is too much for you, send the would-be martial artists to the backyard or basement.

An Unfortunate Trend

Our American lifestyles have changed considerably, even in the last three decades, and the increase in obesity among children reflects these changes. Obesity among children six to eleven has increased by 54 percent since the 1960s, according to a 1987 study by the Harvard School of Public Health. By 1989, only 32 percent of children ages six to seventeen met minimum standards for cardiovascular fitness, flexibility, and abdominal and upper body strength, in contrast to 43 percent who met those standards in 1981. A lack of exercise is a very significant player in this total picture. It's a vicious cycle: Overweight people are less physically fit, so they have less energy, and as a result, they do less. It is essential to help your child break this pattern.

Your child may be unaware of just how little exercise she is getting. When I meet with kids, they often overestimate the amount of physical activity they engage in regularly. "I walk home from the bus stop every day," an eleven-year-old girl told me recently. Her mother was quick to point out that the bus stop was only a block from home. But kids today count even one block of walking as exercise.

Gym class may occur only once or twice a week, yet that's what kids consider their exercise, even though it may amount to only about twenty minutes of moving around by the time they change into gym uniforms, pick teams, and select their equipment. What's worse, gym class may consist of watching films about basketball or other sports without any physical activity at all. After-dinner street play is a thing of the past: Kids no longer run around together, burning off those extra calories and having unsupervised fun. Even the most mundane actions have been taken over by electronics: We drive the kids home from school, open car windows automatically, push the electronic garage door opener, use the remote control to turn on the television. When someone calls, we answer the portable phone at our side, without having to run for the telephone. And instead of biking to the library, our kids use the Internet to research their homework. As a culture, we are less active than ever. And there are many kids who get so little exercise that just walking to the mailbox is a big deal.

Parental Guidance Suggested

There's no doubt about it. With the decline in supervised fitness opportunities in school, it falls to us as parents to make sure our kids acquire the exercise habit. If fitness is a regular part of your life, your children will just assume it's a part of their lives too. For a long time now, parents have been told that the best way to encourage reading is to be a reader. Children learn what's important to you by watching what you do. The same thing is true for exercise. Seeing parents enjoy exercise sends a strong message. It doesn't even have to seem like exercise. Teach your child to be active. Just as you teach your kids to brush their teeth every morning, or to keep themselves clean, teach them to keep their bodies fit. Make fitness a part of life.

As a parent, there are three ways you can promote fitness in your children. First of all, you have to make sure there are opportunities for regular activity: The right clothes and equipment; access to a park, playground, yard, or court; enough free time to participate; and friends to play with. If your neighborhood is safe and traffic is not a threat, encourage them to walk. But not everyone has this option, so you may have to be creative. Second, you must see yourself as a role model: Your child learns from you. If physical fitness is a priority for you, a regular part of your life, your child will get the message. Does this mean that Mom goes to the aerobics studio every day and the kids should do the same? Definitely not. But let them see activity as a regular part of life, something you enjoy rather than dread. Something that is important to you.

And finally, participate with your kids. Go for a parent-child bike ride. Walk the dog together. Go ice skating. Your child will skate longer if you are out there skating with her. You'll get more participation when you go along. Parental support is an essential part of establishing a regular fitness routine for children.

If they see that you consider fitness important, it will mean something to them. Attend games and field days. Arrive early to pick your child up from dance class so you can watch. If your child joins a sports team or takes lessons, be there often to show your interest. Plan a canoe trip or family hike. (Variety will keep your child active. The more activities, the better.) Your interest means a lot to her. If scheduling is impossible, make other plans together. Active vacation packages are available, and family resorts have programs that appeal to all ages.

Make fitness a part of your family life. If your little one watches from the sidelines as an older sibling plays soccer, you can bet he will be eager to get out there when his time comes. Practicing sports skills together is a great way to spend some family time. Everyone can get involved.

As for day-to-day activities, I've found that kids don't mind doing something, such as walking to the store, when there is a purpose in mind—buying stamps, selecting a new comic book—whatever will focus attention on the destination and not the effort it takes to get there. Don't fall prey to your child's request that you drive rather than walk. A fifteen-minute walk to the park is something kids can get used to.

Hidden Benefits

Supporting your child's interest in fitness has benefits beyond just promoting her good health. For one thing, spending time together allows you to get to know your child during these activities. So often, our kids give us one-word answers to our well-intentioned "How was your day?" But a conversation on the way to or from somewhere, or as you are doing something else, is a more comfortable place for things to come up.

As a participant in your child's fitness regimen, you too can benefit. Why not take advantage of your child's newly active lifestyle to make some changes yourself?

There are other rewards in it for you, too. For one thing, it's fun to spend time playing with your child. Siblings, too, develop special relationships as they participate in physical activities together. Even a five-year-old is old enough to start biking with the family. Begin early in life, and your child will enjoy fitness activities for years to come. Your kids are much more likely to participate when the whole family is involved.

Of course, the reality is that of all this takes time and energy, and trying to fit exercise into your schedule and budget is sometimes hard. You have to pick and choose: The investment in a basketball hoop for your driveway may be worth it to you. Making plans to go to the park with your kids is another kind of investment—of time. But even busy parents can find half an hour. It's not easy. I won't kid you. But make the time. It's worth it.

The Greatest Gift

One of the greatest gifts you can give your child is to help him grow up to be physically active. It really is a gift: Exercise is so important for your child's body, helping to prevent disease and control weight. And it improves his emotional health, too, building self-confidence and saving him from the misery

---

FAST FACT: Don't Let "Natural" Products Fool You

Healthy-sounding snacks may not always be low-calorie or low-fat. One ounce of each of these snacks contains:

regular potato chips	150 calories	10 gm. fat
Hain Carrot Chips	160 calories	9 gm. fat
Terra Chips (root vegetable mixture)	140 calories	7 gm. fat
Sweet Potato Chips	140 calories	7 gm. fat

of being unfit and overweight. If your child continues the exercise habit into adulthood, she has a head start on staying healthy, having fun, making friends, and combating some of the effects of aging. By giving your child an interest in fitness, you are giving your child a happier, healthier future.

Beware the Sports Drink!

Gatorade and other sports drinks are marketed as athletic essentials, but don't let this marketing ploy become license for your child to down a quart of extra calories.

Here are the facts:

- Unless you're a marathon runner, enduring sustained activity for three hours without replenishing your fluids, any electrolytes your body loses through perspiration are easily replaced by normal food consumption throughout the day.
- Water is the best thirst quencher and the healthiest, lowest-calorie choice.

Note: Drinking water before and during an activity is important, particularly in hot weather. Give your child one or two 8-ounce glasses of water before exercising, and as much water as he or she wants during an activity. Don't believe the old wives' tale that drinking during physical activity is bad for the body.

8

When to Say no to a "Hungry" Child:

A Survival Guide for Holidays, Special Occasions, and Daily Temptations

Many parents have great difficulty with the idea of restricting their child's eating. How do you deny food to your hungry child? After all, food is nourishment, nourishment is nurturing, and nurturing is love. How can you deny your child love?

Anthony, age eight, already weighed 112 pounds. An only child, he was very much indulged by his extended family. All his life, this little boy ate anything and everything he wanted. His parents never said no. They allowed him every high-fat treat he loved, even though they were aware of his weight problem. By the time they brought him to see me, he had been having a lot of trouble with the kids at school and was quite unhappy.

At Easter, eleven-year-old Elizabeth's grandmother brought her a basket filled with chocolate candy as she had done every year. When Elizabeth refused to eat the candy, her grandmother urged her to have some—even if only a little bit at a time. Later, Elizabeth told her father, "It's too hard! Don't give me all that chocolate!" Together, they asked her grandmother not to give Elizabeth candy anymore, but to find another gift instead.

Setting limits is a real challenge. But one of the most loving things a parent can do for an overweight child is to set some limits. Sure, the child may protest; few of us have Elizabeth's willpower to "just say no" to extra calories. In time, however, the family of an overweight child can settle into a rhythm that allows for real give-and-take and, ultimately, progress. Still, it can be hard to find this rhythm.

Why is limit setting with food so difficult? There are many reasons. First, parents fear they will deprive their child of some essential nutrient by restricting the foods he eats, even though a child who is overweight is getting more than enough of what he needs to grow. Second, parents are afraid that drawing attention to overweight will cause emotional problems such as eating disorders or low self-esteem. Third, parents who are themselves overweight may have difficulty asking their child to act with more discipline than they can muster. Fourth, parents may genuinely believe that more is better: Three bananas are better than one, eight glasses of milk are better than three, and so on. Fifth, it's a natural inclination: Parents enjoy nurturing their children, giving them life, giving them pleasure, fulfilling their needs. And finally, a strong-willed child can make it very difficult for any parent to say no, as most of us probably have experienced. It's simply easier to say yes. The time has come to set aside these underlying conflicts and recognize that the very best thing you can do for your child is set

---

FAST FACT: **Not All Pasta Sauces Are Alike**

One ½-cup serving of pasta sauce varies in calories, depending on the brand:

Ragu Light Tomato and Herb	50 calories
Del Monte Chunky Italian Herb	60 calories
Classico Tomato and Basil	60 calories
Contadina Fresh Four Cheese	320 calories
Prego Traditional	150 calories
Progresso Alfredo	310 calories

some limits and in time teach your child to accept these limits and make them a part of daily living.

A Part of Parenting

In truth, setting limits with food is no different from setting limits in other areas of your child's life—when she goes to bed at night, how much television she can watch, whether she can spend the night at a friend's house, and so on. From the time you first bring your child home, you are constantly making judgment calls. Do I call the doctor now, or see how the baby feels later? Do I take my son's phone privileges away as punishment, or restrict his plans this weekend? Should I go in and speak to the teacher immediately, or wait and see how she handles the situation? Sometimes, your family's "house rules" are enough to go on. But there are countless situations that require individual, on-the-spot decisions. That's what being a parent is all about.

Food choices are no different. Over the course of your child's life, you will make thousands of decisions about how to nourish her. As your child gets older, the kinds of decisions you make will change. The one constant is attitude: Being flexible, open to compromise, can prevent battles and lead to true cooperation within the family as your child grows. The Plan in Chapter 6 offers guidelines for day-to-day living. This chapter, however, is for all those exceptions: when your child is at school, at camp, at a friend's house, or at a restaurant with or without you. It also offers strategies for holiday eating, when the temptations of the season can get the best of us. In these situations, you can't limit choices to what's on the Plan and must negotiate to keep your child happy for the moment while still maintaining his or her overall weight goals.

Limit setting is hard. But your child needs your help to keep him from overeating, and setting limits on what he eats is the way to do this. Remember, your child is not on a diet, so you are not asking him *not* to eat. Eating is a good thing. Your child needs to eat. And enjoying food is part of childhood.

Being clever about how you feed your child will keep your family life on an even keel as you move ahead with this lifestyle change.

This chapter contains all my favorite solutions for the situations in which parents have trouble saying no. Naturally, not all of these solutions are my own ideas—over the years, many of the best strategies have been supplied by parents of patients and by patients themselves. Over time, you will come up with a few of your own creative ideas as well.

As you will see, the general principles are these:

• **Give your child a choice.** You're the parent, so you set the boundaries—but let your child have some input. Even young children need the chance to choose either a soda or a dessert, a cookie now or some candy later, a lollipop at the bank or an afternoon snack.

• **Set some financial boundaries.** At the candy store, the pool snack bar, or when the ice cream truck arrives, tell your child she can have a certain amount to spend–and that's it. Fifty cents buys lots of penny candy; a dollar is enough for an ice treat (but, luckily, not enough for a high-calorie ice cream cookie sandwich or similar indulgence!). Set an amount based on what things really cost, a reasonable amount that gives your child a few items to choose from. This strategy gives you a way to set limits without making your child feel bad by bringing up the topic of overweight. And it lets you off the hook: It's torture for a parent to go up to an ice cream truck and have to say no to the first five things a child requests.

• **Negotiate.** Giving in occasionally may stave off binges, secret or otherwise. Your child will no doubt try to talk you into changing your standards. She wants fifty cents for candy every day, and you've said only twice a week? Giving in even a little— say, going to three times a week on alternate weeks—can keep her from feeling resentful enough to sneak candy and calories later.

• **Let kids be kids.** This is the cornerstone of my program: Let your child have a happy childhood, with all the pleasures of eating that a happy childhood suggests. If you follow this program, an unexpected indulgence here or there will not be a problem.

The larger lesson here is compromise: Your child should learn that no one can have everything he wants all the time. That's a basic lesson of life, and when you think of it as such, it's not so hard to hold to as a parent. Your child is not entitled to unlimited amounts of candy every day after school. You give your child limits, but you also give your child choices within those limits. There are many ways to compromise without making your child feel oppressed or deprived or resentful. I think the trick is to give him some level of choice in advance. Don't say, "No dessert—because you drank that soda with dinner." Let him know in time to make an informed decision. Before dinner, announce, "I'm not buying appetizers and desserts for everyone, so you can choose which to have." And he can understand that nobody gets everything every time. After all, you would never go into a toy store and agree to buy anything and everything your child loads into your arms. Instead you say, "One toy for five dollars or under," or "Add anything else you want to your birthday wish list."

The section that follows contains a laundry list of situations and solutions. As you read through them, you will no doubt think of similar situations and ways you might solve them.

Family Matters

When we talk about setting limits, parents often ask: "What about the rest of the family?" They find it hard to imagine forcing the entire family to cut back simply because one child is overweight. So do I, and I don't recommend it. It's best to prepare a single family meal rather than special-ordering for the overweight child. The good news is that my menus will appeal to all. Part of supporting your child through his struggle with overweight is learning to live without some of the high-calorie treats you yourself love. "Why should I give up my favorite cookies? I'm not the one with the weight problem!'' I have heard comments like this over the years. Do it for your child. If you must, keep cookies in your desk drawer at work. Have a candy bar in the car on your way home. Slip out quietly alone for an ice cream. But don't tempt your child by keeping forbidden foods in the house.

If you feel as though you are depriving your normal-weight kids, find other times during the day to provide them with a few "extras"—as you run errands, for example, or in their lunches. Just as you make time for your children's different needs—help with homework, rides to tennis or dance lessons—you can find a way to give them the additional calories they need and can afford when your overweight child is elsewhere. Where normal-weight siblings are concerned, the little ones are at home more, so you can indulge them when you're alone together; your older kids are more independent and have more opportunity for snacking on their own. It's not as hard to make these adjustments as you might think. After all, if your spouse had a high cholesterol level, you'd be able to work around it. You'd take the kids to an ice cream parlor rather than bring ice cream home. You'd try some recipes without red meat. Think of low-calorie eating like any other special dietary need.

As for allowing your other children to order in restaurants with all-you-can-eat abandon, forget it. Nobody—whether overweight or not—needs appetizers *and* main courses *and* fries *and* sodas *and* dessert. As budget-conscious parents know, there are other reasons to set limits for *all* your kids: Restaurants are expensive, after all. The principle that you just can't have everything you want all the time holds for all family members in all situations. Keeping this in mind helps to keep you from shining an uncomfortable spotlight on your overweight child, who may feel guilty if she believes she is the only reason her brothers and sisters have to do without a soft drink or skip dessert.

A united parental front is essential to the success of this

Plan. Whether you are married or divorced, you should agree to maintain the Plan's continuity to the fullest extent possible, for the sake of your child. Parents who are divorced should be sure to select activities for visitation that focus on something other than food—which may be easier on weekends than on weeknights. Whatever the case, as parents, you should discuss your dietary disagreements in private. Now, more than ever, your child needs you to be responsible and supportive. Allowing your child to cheat when the other parent isn't looking hurts his chances for success.

Each situation is different. But you see the many possibilities in these examples. I invite you to devise your own creative solutions. See what works best for your family, and be open to new strategies as your children get older.

The Danger Zone: Problems and Solutions

School and Day Care

School lunches: If Monday is Pizza Day, your child will probably want to participate. And if all the other kids eat two slices, then she will want two slices, too. I say, let her. But if two slices are more than your child's Plan allows, then have her com-

---

FAST FACT: **Sandwich Spreads Calorie Countdown**

In a ¼ cup serving of these popular salads, prepared with mayonnaise:

egg salad	178 calories
chicken salad	104 calories
tuna salad (light tuna in water)	74 calories
shrimp salad	71 calories

Source: Food Consumption Survey, Nutrient Database, U.S. Department of Agriculture, 1994.

pensate for the extra calories by giving up something later in the day. Similarly, if all the kids get dessert and juice with lunch, your child will want both, too. The solution? Ask her to alternate, having dessert one day and juice the next.

School events: If they're passing out the cupcakes for a class party, let your child get in line. Don't ask her—or her teacher—to restrict treats. Being different is the last thing your child wants. Keep tabs, but be reasonable and forgiving. Your child can always make up for it by giving up a snack later.

The snack trade: Children trade snacks and lunch items at school, and it's hard for parents to regulate. Trading starts much earlier than you think, and it is a normal part of socialization. So don't tell your child not to trade snacks. Let him socialize normally. Forbidding your child to trade snacks can cause peer rejection, and often the items traded are no better or worse than what you sent along yourself.

Day care: Encourage your day-care provider to serve low-calorie snacks, but don't single your child out. If cookies and juice are the snack of choice, then so be it. But factor the day-care snack into the overall plan for eating.

Recreation

The movies: Buy your candy elsewhere first. Movie theater portions are enormous; a movie box of m&m's is a third or more larger than the average pack. Allow extra time to stop, get a smaller serving, and take it in with you. Your kids won't mind, because the selection is greater at stores than at the movies! The theaters, however, generally prefer that you buy their snack foods, so be discreet.

Some theaters offer bins of selected Raisinets, gummy bears, and other candies that allow movie-goers to mix their own treats. You can select lower-calorie items over higher-fat choices and buy a smaller amount.

Incidentally, movie theater popcorn is notoriously high in fat—with or without butter. I don't recommend it, but if you must, look for air-popped, or at the very least, a small-size bag.

After the game: It's great that your child is exercising and making friends, so don't single him out by denying him the fun of after-game snacks and parties. When parents bring snacks and drinks, let her enjoy them. And never tell her in front of her friends that she should limit her intake; that can really be embarrassing. Later on, you can suggest she make up for those extra calories by skipping a snack or dessert. "Well, since you had some doughnuts after the game, how about saving your cookies for tomorrow?" It can all balance out with a little planning.

Group activities: Everyone's going out for ice cream after a music recital. Should you exclude your child? Absolutely not. But don't go overboard. A single dip with a few sprinkles is plenty!

Summer Camp: Plenty of kids gain weight at camp. Unlimited servings of high-calorie foods, the chance to take crafts or computers instead of canoeing or swimming, and secret stashes of candy in the possession of generous friends often result in weight gain.

When making summer plans with your overweight child, choose day camps or overnight camps where kids are on the go, with more outdoor activities than indoor. Whether it's day or sleep-away camp, your kids are on their own when it comes to food. I think they'll be fine as long as they are required to be active.

Camp activities are hard to monitor. You might be thinking tennis, but your child could choose ceramics. Even "athletic" camps can fool you: You may have visions of your son running up and down the field at soccer camp, when he's actually spending all afternoon in a goalie clinic. Watch out also for camps that allow kids to choose too many sit-down activities. Look for a variety of activities to balance out the day.

Beverage intake at camp usually needs some limits. Buffet-style dining and visiting the canteen—the snack bar where kids can get candy, sometimes nightly—can be other problem areas. Believe me, the pounds can add up quickly when your child is away from home. One six-year-old boy I know gained four pounds during the last five months of the school year, and gained another four pounds in one month of camp! So don't ignore the idea of buffet strategy; your child needs to learn it.

To make an informed camp choice for your overweight child, consider these suggestions.

- There are many camps that offer outdoor activities of all kinds for beginners, so don't let skill level be a stopper. Find a camp that welcomes inexperienced campers.
- Talk to the camp director about the camp's philosophy, and when possible, observe campers in action: Do counselors allow kids to skip swimming or hiking simply because they ask to? It's best to find a camp where kids are expected to participate in all activities. Do what you can to make sure your child will have an active summer. I'm not advocating competitive athletics for a nonathlete, just an environment where getting up and moving around is expected from everyone.
- Overweight kids sometimes try to beg off from physical activities, so talk to your child beforehand about participation. Let your child know that taking part in activities is a part of going to camp.
- Find out about food service, and beware of the open buffet; kids overindulge without even thinking about it. If buffet is the only option, encourage your child to have first helpings only—no seconds or thirds.
- Inquire about the rules and how well kids follow them. Does a no-candy rule stick, or do kids sneak? (I know of

one popular day camp where kids actually make a game of sneaking candy in and hiding it in their lockers.) You need to follow the rules, too. Camps have their own reasons for limiting snacks and care package contents, so don't disregard them. There are plenty of treats during camp itself.

Ask questions, talk to your child, and make your camp decision carefully. It's not enough to assume that camp equals increased activity. It's not that simple anymore, and kids know they can get out of things by becoming "squeaky wheels." But don't be discouraged. I see just as many kids who participate fully, enjoy themselves, and end the summer without weight gain! The key is participation.

Weight-loss camps: Parents often ask me about weight-loss camps for their kids. I feel that there are positives and negatives associated with these camps. They can provide a supportive environment in which overweight children can have fun, make friends, and feel comfortable and accepted. The problem is, managing a weight problem in a tightly controlled environment is generally easier than doing so back at home. I've known many kids who have rapidly gained back the weight they lost over the summer upon returning to their usual routines. So consider carefully the best option for your child. If she asks to attend a weight-loss camp, fine. Otherwise, a regular camp that emphasizes outdoor activities would be another option, providing your child with new, calorie-burning interests she can pursue throughout the year.

Your Social Animal

Play dates: I think it overburdens the other parent to expect her to keep an eye on your child's food intake during play-dates. And it would also be unfair to your child. Talk to your child first and prepare him for the decision making that will take place. But then, whatever happens happens. Not to worry—half of your child's play dates will be at your home, where it will be easier for you to watch what goes on.

Birthday parties: Birthday parties may well be the biggest social events in the life of your child, who may attend several in one weekend alone. You probably won't be on hand to guide your child at a birthday party, so there are a few things you should consider. For one thing, the days of mere cake and ice cream are gone. Most birthday parties today involve a lot of food, from snacks to full meals with candy and dessert. Kids typically go home with treats, too. These "goodie bags" filled with candy should be dealt with much the same as the Halloween trick-or-treat bag (see page 174 for more details).

What can you do? Doling out a bit each day until it's gone is a good way to deal with this. Don't let your child eat the whole bag of candy that afternoon. Not only has she already consumed enough extras at the party, but she also needs to work these treats carefully into the Eating Plan. Perhaps she could skip the afternoon snack, or both afternoon and evening snacks, depending on how many extras she has consumed.

Family parties and celebrations: Throughout the year, there are gatherings at which food is the focus: Weddings, birthday parties, Bar Mitzvahs, and celebrations of all kinds are a challenge for the child who is trying to control his weight. Here are some tips to make things easier for your child:

- Talk to your child ahead of time. Decide how the party food will fit in with the overall plan for that day and come up with a game plan for enjoying what's offered.
- Don't arrive hungry. A hungry child will feel like eating a whole plateful of finger food, which is generally high in calories. Instead, go ahead and serve breakfast and lunch and a snack, and then figure out whether the party will serve as dinner or not. You can even have a light dinner before the party to stave off hunger.

- Do not call attention to your child if she is overeating at the party. This is humiliating. Instead, wait until after the party to discuss ways to compensate by skipping snacks or having a light supper rather than a full dinner later.
- If there is an array of desserts, ask your child to choose one item only, or to have just a sliver of a few different desserts.

Don't expect perfection. Parties are filled with temptation. But as long as you factor parties into your Plan, they can remain a part of your son's or daughter's childhood. You'll soon discover your own solutions. I know adults who pour water on their plates when they're finished so they won't keep nibbling, or eat a meal at home before going out for an evening. Who's to say some similar techniques wouldn't work for kids? Experiment with my suggestions, make some of your own, and see what works best for your child.

Sleep-overs: Part of the fun of sleeping over at a friend's house is the late-night snacking. Everyone probably has fond memories of "raiding the refrigerator" or making popcorn to eat while watching an old movie. These days, renting videos is the norm, and kids always want to eat as the drama unfolds. When your child has an overnight guest, make sure you offer snacks from the Product Guide and take any extra snacks into account when planning the day's eating. Dance contests or other physical activities are a good way to get kids up and moving while taking the focus off of food.

What about when your child spends the night at a friend's house, where make-your-own sundaes are the featured eating event of the evening, rounded out with chips beforehand and hot chocolate afterward? Being with other kids the whole night long only encourages the eating.

Talk with your child ahead of time. Your child wants to succeed at weight control, but she's likely to be worried about the temptations and will probably be glad for the chance to work on some coping strategies. Brainstorm together about what the problems might be and discuss some solutions. For example:

- When choosing between chips and popcorn, popcorn is the better choice. Baked pretzels are another excellent alternative.
- Making a sundae doesn't have to mean a three-scoop banana split. One scoop of ice cream with some sprinkles and a little syrup is plenty. (Nuts are high in fat and calories, so you may wish to discourage your child from choosing them.)
- Candy, chips, *and* cookies? Either choose just one, or have only a little of each.
- Agree on one serving of flavored beverage—a canned drink, for instance. After that's gone, encourage water.
- Extra exercise the day of the sleep-over and the day after can help undo the "damage."

Shopping

The grocery store: We all fall prey to our kids' "grocery store gimmes." We're in a rush, they're whining, and everybody's tired. Young children, in particular, become tiny dictators from their shopping basket perches. "I want chips." "I want cookies." "I want ice cream." "Mommy, can we get some of that?" "Mommy, how about some of these?" It shouldn't be so hard to say no. The solution? Plan ahead. Make a shopping list and ask for your children's help in selecting products along the way. Show them the options you have chosen and let them pick. "Which cereal would you like?" Do the same thing with snacks. Take the Product Guide with you and use it.

Going to the store only after a meal when nobody's hungry is a great idea. But in most households, that's a lot easier said than done. Most people get to the grocery whenever they can work it in, and that means dealing with the inevitable gimmes.

It may be best to just give your child a snack as you begin your shopping: That way, she's satisfied for the time being and you can get on with your shopping.

Checkout lines. Aaaagh! We know stores do it on purpose: Invite us in to shop, let us work up an appetite, and then tempt us. And not just in grocery stores! Where I live, even the car wash sells candy. The beauty lies in making this final destination work for you: Promise your child that if he or she cooperates, you will buy a treat from the checkout display. Then offer Life Savers or mints—and leave the Kit Kats and Milky Ways for someone else. Or, if there is a countertop box of miniature candies such as Peppermint Patties or Tootsie Rolls, buy a few of these instead (they have fewer calories than their full-sized counterparts.) With a strategy in mind, you can avoid the tired tantrum of the treat-deprived while maintaining the plan you have put in place.

Incidentally, some grocery stores have candy-free checkout lines to help us all resist temptation.

The shopkeeper's candy dish: It's nice to live in a community where everyone is so friendly that your child is offered a treat wherever you go. It can get tricky. A candy cane at the cleaner's is no big deal. Let your child say thank you and accept the treat. A handful of lollipops at the gas station? Again, let your child say thanks. Let the child enjoy one lollipop right then and save the others for another occasion. Cider and doughnuts at the bank? Sure, one cup of cider and one doughnut. Moderation is the key here. Your child should be allowed to enjoy these perks of childhood! But you can set limits. Go with the flow as much as you can, but watch out for overflow!

Out and About

In a restaurant: When you go out to eat, your kids may think they've got you. They know you won't want to get into a big battle, so they may push you to allow them to take "all you can eat" to new heights. But applying the basic principles of give and take can work wonders here. They can't have everything. So you let them choose: soda or dessert? Fries or an appetizer? There are limits, but your children have a choice within those limits. (Personally, I believe these limits are appropriate whether there is a weight problem or not. Parents today often buy too much for their children, and a good deal always remains uneaten.) Sharing is another great solution:

Dining Out

Americans are eating out more than ever, and our habits at restaurants are different from our habits at home. We usually make worse choices when faced with a restaurant menu, consuming more food and more calories than we need or may even want just because we're out enjoying ourselves. Here are some tips for successful restaurant dining:

- Select all restaurants carefully. Avoid restaurants where everything is fried.
- Limit fast-food meals to one or two per month.
- Make a habit of asking for an extra plate and splitting a single entrée.
- Don't be a "clean-plater." Serving sizes these days are bigger than ever, so consider eating half of your serving and taking the other half home in a doggie bag.
- Choose a drink or dessert, not both.
- Order a single appetizer for all the kids to share, rather than one per child.
- Ask for salad dressings, sauces, and toppings on the side—then use them sparingly.
- Have dessert at home—and select from your plan.
- Stay away from all-you-can-eat buffets. If you can't avoid them, limit the meal to first helpings only, no seconds or thirds.
- Beware of these high-fat buzz words: batter-dipped, breaded, creamy, crispy, flaky, and fried. Instead, look for: grilled, poached, roasted, steamed, or marinara.

One soda and one dessert to share with a brother or sister. A single order of fries for two. And let them work it out. (Sharing is another important life lesson.)

Away from home: As your children grow, they have more opportunities to eat outside your home, and you have less control. Limit setting therefore takes on a different flavor for the older child. Going out to lunch with friends, for example, is a calorie risk. Again, a good way to control how much food your child buys and eats is the pocketbook. A few dollars is enough to get a slice of pizza and a small drink; any more could lead to a larger soda, an extra topping, and a candy bar. Ten dollars is too much. Giving him a reasonable amount of money is an easy way to set a limit.

What'll It Be?

When dining out, encourage your child to select from among these lower-calorie menu choices:

FAST FOOD

regular hamburger—skip the cheese and "special" sauce
small fries—to share
grilled (not breaded) chicken breast sandwich
salad with chicken chunks
garden salad (go easy on the dressing!)

ITALIAN

pasta with red sauce
pasta with clam sauce
bread (no butter!)
minestrone soup
pasta e fagioli soup (pasta and bean soup)
green salad (dressing on the side!)

CHINESE

wonton soup (But forget those fried noodles—hand them back to the waiter!)
chicken, beef, or shrimp with vegetables
white or brown rice (not fried)
fortune cookie—easy to enjoy at only 35 calories

MEXICAN

gazpacho soup
salsa—as a food topping (don't dig into those high-fat chips!)
bean or chicken enchilada
bean or chicken burrito
chicken or vegetable fajita
yellow or white rice
ceviche

DINER

baked chicken—remove the skin
sandwich—to share (diner sandwiches are often huge!)
baked potato (watch the toppings!)
salad or vegetable
no dessert—until later, when you get home (diner desserts are also huge!)

The ice cream truck: Oh, those ringing bells! Pavlov's children—and my own—simply *have* to buy an ice cream when they hear that familiar sound. (And parents often become nostalgic as they remember their own ice-cream truck days.) But what if your child has already had a snack that afternoon? Let her buy the ice cream (again, use money limits to control choices), but have her store it in the freezer for her after dinner snack or the next day; if she really wants it "now," negotiate for her to forgo her snack later. Again, hearing "yes, but" is much more tolerable to your child than hearing "no"—and another argument is avoided.

Special treats: All parents enjoy giving their kids treats from time to time, and you don't need to stop doing so just because your child is overweight. There are a number of items you can use in a pinch if you know what is low in calories and offer it as an occasional extra treat. A Tootsie Pop, for instance, is lower in calories than a candy bar. When you step out of the gas station with a surprise lollipop, your child will be thrilled, you'll be the hero, and nobody is the wiser, though the calorie count is low. Another effective trick with younger children is to buy five or six individual candies—one-bite caramels or individually wrapped hard candies. Kids love the feeling of a whole handful of candy, and you avoid the calorie blowout of a jumbo candy bar. Consider surprising them with a comic book, hair clips, or a pair of crazy socks as an alternative—surprises don't always have to be food.

At Home

Leftovers: Holidays and parties can create an abundance of remnants—chips and dips, cakes, cheeses. I advise getting rid of as much as possible to avoid temptation. Even putting it in the freezer is risky, because older children are quite adept at thawing out and reheating. Instead, send care packages home with your guests or take some to a neighbor. Keeping a day or two's worth of leftovers is plenty for your family.

Dessert: Ask a child if he or she wants dessert and the answer will always be yes. It rounds out the meal and makes the child feel satisfied. Dessert is one of the pleasures of childhood. Rather than pass out the high-cal brownies, try some other options, such as a low-calorie fudge pop or a single decorated holiday cookie.

Travel

On the road: Pack your own meals and drinks and have a picnic or eat in the car. Picnicking along the way helps limit fast-food cravings, and it's a nice way to break up the trip. Take along a to-go box of lower-calorie snacks as well.

In the air: Airplane peanuts are fattening, and kids will probably still be hungry after eating them, so pack some favorite low-calorie snacks to keep complaints to a minimum. These days, many airlines are "no frills," providing a boxed snack or no food at all—all the more reason to pack your own. Even if it's a meal flight, I still recommend packing your meal. Your sandwiches will no doubt be tastier as well as better for you. Take along some games or books so your kids won't get bored and ask for food.

On vacation: Whenever possible, stay somewhere that has a kitchenette where you can prepare some meals yourself. The room rate may be slightly higher, but you'll save on food costs—*and* save calories! Family resorts and cruises with all three meals included are a trap for anyone with a weight problem. Whether you mean to or not, you end up thinking, "Well, I've already paid for it. I might as well eat it!" If you have to restrict your child as others go back for seconds and thirds, you are bound to have a very tense vacation. Compensate for the extra calories by increasing your activities—easy to do in most vacation areas. For a change of pace, try an adventure vacation, going hiking, camping, or rafting. These trips are great for families, giving them the chance to have fun together and stay active!

At Grandma and Grandpa's

"We're grandparents! We can bring candy if we want to!" More than any other relatives, grandparents love to spoil the children they love. Oftentimes, a talk with Grandma or Grandpa will help, but they may also decide that your child's weight problem is something you can deal with when they are not around. If they visit only occasionally, the problem may be minimal and best overlooked. But if the grandparents are a regular part of the household, you should try to enlist their help and support.

With Baby-Sitters

Communicate your concerns and provide the Plan-approved snacks your child prefers. Let the sitter know which snacks are okay and how many to dole out. There's no need to go into great detail about the Plan with a sitter who comes only occasionally. Regular sitters or nannies, however, should be enlisted to keep your child on track. In any event, making it easy for the sitter makes it easier for you.

FAST FACT: Popular Popcorns

Calories vary widely when it comes to popcorn. Compare these 3-cup servings:

Pop Secret Lite Butter microwave popcorn	70 calories
Jolly Time Natural Lite microwave popcorn	72 calories
Pop Secret By Request Natural microwave pop-corn	65 calories
Pop Secret By Request Butter microwave pop-corn	65 calories
Orville Redenbacher Smart Pop microwave pop-corn	40 calories
Orville Redenbacher Natural Light microwave popcorn	60 calories
Smart Food Butter ready-to-eat popcorn	150 calories
Smart Food Plain & Simple ready-to-eat popcorn	150 calories
Jiffy Pop Lite Butter microwave popcorn	120 calories
Vic's Corn Popper Butter ready-to-eat popcorn	180 calories
Newman's Own Old Style Picture Show Natural microwave popcorn	146 calories

Source: Environmental Nutrition, July 1994.

Month-to-Month Tips for Happy Holidays

Parents are usually enthusiastic about my plan—until a holiday approaches. Then they panic. "The day-to-day routine of eating is one thing, but what about holidays? Is it really possible to allow my child to enjoy holiday treats? Or should I downplay certain holidays so my child can stick to the Plan?"

Here's the remarkable thing about this program for eating: Your child can stick to the Plan and still enjoy holiday treats! I would never want to deprive a child of the fun of the holidays, and food is definitely a part of that fun! True, it's tougher to handle the program at holiday time, but you can work around these challenges by being creative. The next section shows you how. Remember to offset those excess holiday calories by seeing that your child gets some exercise every day—school's out, maybe you're home from work, so make the most of it! Take a walk. Go for a bike ride. Play some ball. And if your child comes through a holiday break holding his own, that's great!

These days, it seems like there is a special occasion for every season, from Halloween to Memorial Day, from Thanksgiving to the Fourth of July—not to mention the countless birthday parties, sleep-overs, wedding receptions, bar mitzvahs, and other events where eating has become the main entertainment. Can your child survive these events? Absolutely! Let's look at a calendar of calorie-busting strategies that will keep your child in the swing of things year round. We start with the school year.

September

After Labor Day, the school year gets under way and your family's schedule changes. Autumn is typically a weight-gaining season because children may be less active than they are in summertime, so the number of calories-out may be lower. The pool closes, camp is over, it gets darker earlier, there's homework to deal with, and it's just not the same. September's not

so bad—the weather's still nice, there are no special temptations—but look out for October!

October

For kids, Halloween is right up there with the winter holidays on the excitement scale. Anticipation builds for weeks:
Stores display Halloween costumes and candy for more than
a month in advance; there may be dishes of candy corn on
shop counters. People get into the spirit, planning parties in
the neighborhood or at school. Don't let your child miss out
on the fun.

Halloween is kids' one chance to do and be whatever they
want, and a brimming bag of trick-or-treat candy is a big part
of the fun. Don't deny your child this thrill. Instead, devise a
strategy ahead of time for dealing with all the treats. Here are
some suggestions:

- Wait until the last minute to buy candy for trick-or-
  treaters. This will limit the temptations at home. The
  longer you have the treats in the house, the more chances
  your child has to dig into them. If you can, buy candy the
  day before Halloween. The stores won't run out.
- Make sure the treats you buy to give away aren't too tempting. If your kids hate coconut, buy Almond Joys. If they
  hate peanuts, choose PayDay bars. Do *not* buy your child's
  favorites. Buy candies they could take or leave.
- Get rid of leftover treats. As the last few trick-or-treaters
  straggle by, go ahead and surprise them by dropping two
  or three or more treats into their bags—until it's all gone.
  Do not keep extras around. Give them to a neighbor or
  relative. Take them to the office if you prefer. But get
  them out of the house.

I want children to enjoy and participate in all holidays. It
would be criminal to take the fun out of Halloween by taking
all of their goodies away or making them stay home. So let
them go trick-or-treating! A few ground rules will make sure

your child enjoys the thrill of Halloween while keeping her from overdoing it:

- Have your child skip the evening snack and instead enjoy something from the trick-or-treat bag that night—either outside during trick-or-treating, or when he gets home.
- When it comes time to sort the loot, tell your child to choose fourteen of her favorite treats from the things that she got. Discard or give away the rest. Those treats will be snack substitutes for the next two weeks, so every day your child can have a treat. Two weeks is plenty of time to extend the holiday. (Smaller kids might only need seven items and one week of this before they forget about it and move on to something else.)

This strategy works because the child gets the chance to choose what he wants. The holiday fun lingers for a few weeks, but there's no "pigging out." And you won't be depriving your child. *No* child needs to eat forty or fifty pieces of candy in a few weeks' time.

Halloween Tricks and Treats

Halloween treats vary in calories, so comparison-shopping is worthwhile. Here is a grab bag of examples:

CANDY	CALORIES
candy corn (¼ cup)	182
Kit Kat (snack size)	170
m&m's (plain, 1 oz.)	135
Hard candy (1 oz.)	106
Snickers (1 snack-size)	100
Hershey's Kisses (3 pieces)	73
Three Musketeers (1 snack size)	70
Nestle Crunch (1 snack size)	50
Reese's Peanut Butter Cup (1 mini)	42
lollipop	22
bubble gum, sugarless (1 piece)	5

- Take control of the remainder. You can either give it away, as you've done with the treats you were passing out Halloween night, or sort through it for Product Guide–approved choices to use as snacks in upcoming weeks. Mini packs of Life Savers—just five in a pack—are a favorite of mine. (A lot of snack-size candies are available only at Halloween time, so it helps to stock up for later use in lunches and as snacks, but hide these treats well!)

November

Thanksgiving is known for its celebration of plenty. But plenty of mashed potatoes, gravy, stuffing, and pie means plenty of extra calories. And if you have your Thanksgiving dinner in your own home, you'll also have plenty of leftovers, which add extras on top of extras. Don't skip this wonderful American tradition. But keep it from turning into a four-day feast by following these tips:

- Prepare a traditional dinner without going overboard on calories. How? Perhaps you could try baked sweet potatoes instead of whipped sweet potato casserole with marshmallow topping, or baked Idaho potatoes instead of creamy mashed potatoes. You can cut calories and still have a satisfying feast.
- Make sure you serve breakfast and lunch. If your child waits all day for dinner, then he will feel justified eating two or three plates full.
- Have your child skip the afternoon and evening snack. In place of those snacks, let your child select a favorite dessert, but make sure it's a moderate portion. Or dole out a sliver of a few different ones to equal one modest piece if it were all put together.
- Treat Thanksgiving dinner like any other meal. Don't act like it's an all-you-can-eat contest. During the meal, let your child have some of everything he or she likes, but not a lot of any one thing. Encourage normal portions for everyone.

- After the main meal, pack it up and move it out. A child who opens the refrigerator and sees an apple pie, a cherry crumb pie, and a pumpkin pie while Mom and Dad are in the den watching football with friends or relatives will find it hard not to help herself to a piece or two. Hold on to just enough leftovers for one more meal and give the rest away. If you have company, put together some care packages to send home with them: A few leftovers are part of the holiday fun, but don't tempt your child with too many available extras.
- Consider organizing a neighborhood football game or family walk. Your children will have fun, get exercise, and you'll have time to cook.

December

The day after Thanksgiving, everything turns holiday. Red and green color the entire world, and Hanukkah gelt, the gold chocolate coins that are a traditional favorite, is offered for sale everywhere. This is when the real challenge begins. If your child can make it through the holiday season just maintaining his current weight, that's success! Plan ahead to help your child meet that goal.

Holiday parties start very early in the season, and there are often a lot of them. The holiday season is different from Thanksgiving because it lasts longer, and there is a great tradition of high-calorie treats associated with it: Christmas cookies, candy canes, holiday chocolates. How do you know when to say yes and when to say no? Here are some suggestions:

- Some Christmas candy is okay. A candy cane is a typical sugary treat, and an appropriate item to substitute for a snack. If a friendly merchant offers one to your child, let him enjoy it instead of a plan-approved snack. Or ask your child to hang on to it until later, perhaps having it as an after-dinner snack. Otherwise, these endless add-ons can add right up. As a parent, try to stay aware of where you are each day in terms of snacks, so you can figure out how to juggle. And if your child's holiday enthusiasm leads him or her to slip one by you, don't worry! The Plan is designed to let things balance out later.

- Don't give up those favorite holiday traditions. Just establish some ground rules. Substitute a few of Grandma's Christmas cookies for a snack item. Compensate for Aunt Rachel's potato pancakes by taking an after-dinner walk. Treat these extras as you have learned to treat the after-practice pizza slice or the classmate's birthday cake.
- Holiday dinners should be like any other. Follow the same guidelines as for Thanksgiving to keep things on track: Limit portion sizes, discard leftovers, and remember to give your child breakfast and lunch to prevent overeating later.
- Offer small toys as stocking-stuffers or in lieu of Hannukah gelt. If you must give sweets, try to select from the Product Guide treats you can allocate as snacks for the week to come.
- If you travel to a warmer climate at holiday time, take advantage by encouraging your child to swim, play tennis, or go for a walk. If you stay where it's cold, look for activities that burn up calories, such as skating, skiing or sledding.
- If you're staying with relatives, talk with your child beforehand about strategies for following the Plan.

January

New Year's Eve isn't a big deal for young children, but New Year's Day often brings open houses and other buffet-style parties where it's hard to pay attention to all your child takes in. The general guidelines for parties will help you manage these festive occasions.

February

Valentine's Day seems to become more and more candy-oriented every year. To keep your child from going calorie crazy, focus instead on things other than food. Younger children may enjoy making their own valentines. And any child will appreciate a special Valentine's Day present such as a book, a game, or a stuffed animal.

School parties may feature candy and cupcakes, so remember to anticipate your child's plans and have her give up a scheduled snack that day. If a goodie bag of treats is part of the festivities, use the same tactic as for Halloween: Count out two weeks' worth of candy and get rid of the rest. Then dole out one treat for each snack time in the days to come.

March

Easter is a tough holiday for anyone who is watching his weight. There is so much emphasis on the seemingly bottomless Easter basket, filled with chocolate bunnies, jelly beans, and countless other treats. Even if you're careful about what goes into a basket at home, your children may receive Easter candy from well-meaning friends and relatives. Find the little tricks that work best with your child:

- Group candies together—whether all of one kind or an assortment—by filling sandwich bags and tying them with festive ribbon. Then allot one bag per snack time. Selecting treats from the Product Guide is always your best bet because you know how they fit in with the overall eating plan.
- Start a new tradition of mixing candy with small, inexpensive toys and other items. Tuck in a cassette tape, tuck in some hair ribbons—be creative and have fun! After all, the thrill of the Easter basket is in the handfuls of goodies it contains, and so long as there's at least some candy, any combination of nonfood treats is likely to bring smiles.

Passover is not as big a problem for weight control because there isn't the same emphasis on sweets. Because of the absence of flour, the baked goods tend to be less appetizing for youngsters. But there are hidden calories everywhere: Every sheet of matzo is 117 calories, about the same as a slice and a half of bread. Spreads like peanut butter, cream cheese, and butter only add to the calories.

April

Springtime holidays may occur during this month instead; follow the same advice as for March.

May

The long Memorial Day weekend kicks off the summer season. Families often celebrate with a picnic or a barbecue, an event that may be repeated throughout the summer. If the barbecue is at your house, you can try the following:

- Serve pretzels or air-popped popcorn as an alternative to potato chips.
- Instead of serving creamy potato salad, toss a green salad with low- or nonfat dressing.
- Grill some chicken instead of the usual hamburgers and hot dogs: Your kids can still put it on a bun if that's part of the fun.

As a picnic guest, you have less control over what is served, but there are still some ways to set limits for your child:

- Volunteer to bring snacks or dessert—which are two calorie-packed summer party selections—and make sure the snacks or dessert you bring are on your approved list.
- Remind your child to stick to one portion: One burger or hot dog, some salad, one cob of corn (without butter, if possible). The picnic supper is still the main meal of the day, so your child need not skimp. But overindulging isn't necessary, either.
- Watch those drinks, which can really add up in calories. Talk things over before the party, and come up with a rule: One canned drink, say, then only water or iced tea. (Brew your own to limit sugar content!)

- Desserts usually abound at these parties. Again, either one choice or a small amount of several, and skip the evening snack later on.
- Help your child burn calories by organizing some children's games so your child will move around: Organize relay races, suggest a game of tag, encourage everyone to head for the playground, or set up a wading pool at the bottom of a sliding board. Become the parent with the answer to "We're bored!" If you like, bring along a soccer ball or volleyball or other equipment to encourage active play.

June

The picnics and cookouts continue. Now that the weather is nice, take advantage by adding physical activity into your child's day. The picnic suggestions for May can help.

July

Fourth-of-July picnics don't have to mean a calorie explosion. The suggestions for May offer calorie-busting tips. And make a day at the beach a day of active fun by walking, playing ball, or jumping waves.

August

Vacations and outings may require a little pre-planning: Choose a vacation spot that gives you control over what your family is eating. The suggestions elsewhere in this chapter offer additional vacation strategies.

A Word of Caution

Trying too hard to control your child's food intake on holidays and during special events can really backfire. If you are too restrictive, your child may rebel by engaging in virtually a one-person pie-eating contest as soon as the dessert buffet is laid. If you focus on finding a balance, your child is far less likely to feel a need to binge. Remember, giving your child choices means a lot. Allowing your child's social life to continue normally sends her the message that you have confidence that she can handle the situation. Offer a few pointers, negotiate and compromise, and everything will work out fine.

As always, never reprimand your child for overeating while at an event. Do not scold, criticize, or draw attention to your child in public. Instead, discuss strategies and tactics in advance and try to anticipate problems, but once the event is under way, it's up to your child, and your interference is a mistake. Trust your child to use his best judgment and you will probably be rewarded.

Some times will be easier than others. A barbecue where the kids run off to play games the minute they're done eating will be easier than a holiday like Thanksgiving, when everyone tends to just sit around and eat. And as you become more familiar with the Plan and Product Guide, it will get easier.

The Pep Talk

As with any endeavor, there will be good days and bad days. For no reason at all, some days just seem easier, and then a hard day arrives. Your child may be tired, anxious about school, a little bored. Just do the best you can, add some extra exercise, and tell yourself—and your child—that tomorrow is another day!

Be Flexible

In every case, all I have done is offer options. It's up to you to discover which work best for your family. You may devise others that are more effective for you. Flexibility is the key. I want what you want: For your child to look forward to and feel good about holidays and other special occasions, and to remember these occasions with joy and happiness, without resenting you for taking the fun out of them. Using these guidelines means you never have to downplay a special event because of overweight. Instead, make a few adjustments later. Help your child to find a way to compensate for the extras that are a wonderful part of childhood.

9

A Teen Guide:

How to Use This Book Yourself to Get Results

If you are a teenager with weight concerns, you are probably interested in trying to get things under control on your own. That's great. You can rest assured that this book contains all you need to know to get started on a plan that will make a big difference in your life. If you've skipped ahead to this chapter, please go back at some point and learn more about weight management by reading the rest of the book.

You're a teenager, which is actually a pretty broad category when it comes to health and fitness. Physically, the body undergoes an extraordinary amount of growth and development during the teen years. In early adolescence, at the onset of puberty, your body requires a great many calories to begin the growth spurt; later, when your physical growth stops and you attain full height, your weight should stabilize. Emotionally, adolescence is a time of increasing independence, and wanting more of a say in what you eat is only natural. So is becoming more concerned about how you look and feel.

You can use this program to help you make good, solid decisions about the foods you consume. Unlike those starvation diets you may have read about—eating nothing but grapefruit, mixing up endless containers of powdered diet shakes— the eating plan I have devised won't interfere with your social life. You can still eat snacks, you can still go out with friends, and you don't have to choose nonfat versions of your favorite foods each time. You can even eat dessert.

But you'll also learn to eat sensibly, by limiting your portion sizes and emphasizing lower-calorie foods. You'll become more active. And that's all there is to it, really: Fewer calories-in and more calories-out equals weight management you can live with.

Your Changing Body

I know, I know. It's hard enough to be an adolescent without having to dwell on all the "wonderful" changes your body is going through. But we do have some ground to cover so you can understand the different needs your body has at different stages of adolescence.

Starting at about age ten, your body is gearing up for some extraordinary developments, and caloric needs can be pretty high. This is why parents often joke about how hard it is to keep food in the house with a teenager around. You may in fact feel hungrier than you used to, and that's perfectly normal. When it comes to managing your weight gain as you grow, the trick is to figure out the magic equation that will get you the calories you need to grow while burning excess calories through exercise. While this growth spurt is happening, be careful: It is still possible to outgain your growth. You can't expect growth to be a cure-all if you're gaining excessively. You

---

FAST FACT: Avoid Cooking with Butter, Margarine, and Oil

Every tablespoon of butter, margarine, and oil contains 100 to 120 calories and 12 to 14 grams of fat. Cook in nonstick pots and pans, and try substituting vegetable oil spray for the real thing: A one- to two-second spray contains only 2 calories and less than 1 gram of fat.

will not outgrow the overweight with which you entered adolescence—at least not without making some significant lifestyle
changes.

For girls, the onset of menstrual periods (around age twelve
and a half) marks the end of rapid growth. A girl may continue
to slowly grow another inch or two over the next year or two,
but seldom more than that. So her caloric intake will need to
slow down at that time or she will start to gain weight excessively. She can no longer count on growth to counteract overeating.

After your growth spurt has stopped, you have attained your
full height, and your weight gain should stabilize. Because you
won't be getting any taller, you don't need to keep eating as
much to keep up with increasing inches. Instead, with your
doctor's help, you want to determine your ideal weight and
eat just enough to fuel your body's daily activities without overeating.

The Teen Lifestyle

As a teen, you are more likely to be eating outside your
home. Schedules get complicated, and eating out may be the
main kind of eating you do. You might pick up breakfast on
the way to school, grab a snack from the vending machine
between classes, head out for fast food with friends at lunch,
and indulge in a slice or two of pizza in the afternoon before
dinner. Those extra calories can really add up, especially once
you've stopped growing taller. At the end of each day, you
have more homework than you used to, and you may develop
the habit of snacking while studying, which means still more
calories.

If you have a job, you may be around food all the time, in
a restaurant, a snack bar, or ice cream parlor. Baby-sitting is
another opportunity for overindulging; after putting the kids
to bed, there's a real temptation to snack until the parents
return (I remember doing this in my baby-sitting days!). Whatever your job, with that extra spending money burning a hole

in your pocket, you'll be able to buy snacks whenever you choose.

You are probably socializing more independently, too. And, let's face it, eating is a big part of the social scene for all of us. You go to the mall and have lunch. You get popcorn and soft drinks at the movies. You have a cookout at the end of softball season. You go on a dinner date. It's just a way of life. Dances, parties, bar and bat mitzvahs, sweet-sixteen celebrations—all of these can center around food, and that's hard when you're watching your weight. Even when there's dancing or some other activity, it's hard to avoid the snack table. Eating is almost incidental to hanging out. You don't want to stick close to home, so you get together with your group of friends and order Cokes and fries or nachos or ice cream, and it can go on for hours. Even if you've been aware of your weight problem for a while, you may have found it hard to "just say no" when you're out with the gang. Chapter 8 talks about ways to set limits when eating out and offers suggestions for handling food on holidays and special occasions. Although these chapters are directed at parents, you can use them yourself as guidelines. Here are some highlights:

- Have a small meal before a party so you're not as eager to dive into the snack trays.
- Limit yourself to one soft drink or other beverage. After that, stick to water.
- If you're asked to bring a snack, select a lower-calorie option from the Product Guide, such as popcorn, pretzels, or even a watermelon.
- At a cookout, team banquet, or other buffet, have first helpings only—no seconds or thirds.
- Bring your own snacks to the movies—and don't be lured by popcorn, which is very high in calories. You could buy a movie snack and eat only part of it, or agree to share with a friend.

If You're a Vegetarian

Over the years, I've treated many teenagers who want to control their weight *and* eat a vegetarian diet. You can have a healthy diet as a vegetarian. But make sure you get enough protein. Some nonmeat alternative sources of protein are milk, cheese, eggs, yogurt, and peanut butter. But be careful: Dairy products and peanut butter are high-fat, high-calorie foods. Go for the low-fat or fat-free milk, cheese, and yogurt, and be very sparing with the peanut butter. You still need to be mindful of your overall calorie intake.

About Alcohol

Teenagers are forbidden by law from drinking alcoholic beverages. But despite the risks—not the least of which is a drunk-driving accident—many still do. I strongly urge any underage person to avoid drinking alcohol. If you are overweight, you have still another reason to abstain: Alcoholic beverages of all kinds—beer, wine, and liquor—are extremely high in calories and are not in any way a part of this Plan.

Your Personal Weight Goals

Social pressures increase during the teenage years. You're attending a larger school, your classmates are starting to separate into different groups or cliques, and you wonder where you fit in. If you suspect you have a weight problem, you may feel quite sensitive. You're not alone.

Many teenagers who come to me have a very specific goal:

I want to lose two dress sizes by the prom in June.
I need to be down fifteen pounds by basketball tryouts.
I should reduce my waist three inches before I leave for college.
I have to drop ten pounds before swim team practice starts.

Sound familiar? The truth is, adults are pretty much the same way. And I tell them exactly the same thing: You didn't put the weight on overnight, and you can't lose it overnight, no matter what they tell you on television. Still, everybody seems to think there's some instant solution.

There *is* a solution, but it isn't instant, so you'll need to make a strong commitment to this new way of life. It won't be as hard as it sounds, because the foods in this plan are pretty much the same foods you already enjoy. But you'll eat less of them. And you'll need to burn more calories with regular exercise.

About Exercise

Team sports are popular with adolescents, and they offer the advantage of regular scheduling: You go to school, you go to sports, and then you go home, without having to make extra time for exercise. If you are into sports, make sure to keep working out in some way even between seasons (walk, jog, or use a workout tape or some sports equipment). The three weeks between football and basketball seasons is plenty of time to lose ground where conditioning is concerned.

If team sports aren't your thing, you're not alone. There are many options for the nonathlete. Physical fitness doesn't mean becoming an expert tennis player. It means improving your strength, endurance, and flexibility. How? By getting at least thirty minutes of good, heart-pumping aerobic exercise three times a week or more. That is what will burn those extra calories. Exercise is also a proven stress buster—and with the pressures of adolescence, it's a safe bet you could use some relief! (In fact, some of you may be consuming extra calories in response to stress, which certainly increases as you reach your teen years.)

Unfortunately, exercise alone is not always enough. You may be on the baseball team, but if you're an outfielder, you're not moving around very much. Soccer can be great exercise, but if you're the goalie, you may or may not be working hard. In these situations, you can supplement with additional exercise.

Whatever activity you choose should keep you breathing rapidly and moving your muscles for thirty minutes or more. Work up a sweat!

If you need a motivator, try enlisting a friend to become your workout buddy. You'll be less likely to cancel plans for a walk or an aerobics class when you know someone's counting on you. And it's always more fun to have a friend along.

Travel Temptations

You're on your own, traveling with a group, participating in an exchange program or summer enrichment program, working as a camp counselor or mother's helper, and your food choices change. Eating opportunities may be limited: Your host family feeds you or you eat meals in a cafeteria or your tour group stops at a fast-food restaurant. Perhaps your opportunities to eat may be unlimited: You're on your own, choosing when and what to eat. Either way, your options are harder to control than when you're at home. Learning to make choices that fit your weight-management goals will keep you on track. Take smaller portions, eat less of the portion you're served, work in extra exercise, fill up on lower-calorie items. (This is an excellent way to deal with restaurant meals in general. Remember, just because they've served it to you doesn't mean you have to clean your plate!)

Off to College

You may have heard about the Freshman Fifteen—the legendary "automatic weight gain" that all new college students are said to endure. How does it happen? Think about it.

***FAST FACT:* Weighing Your Breakfast Options**

A low-fat waffle with 1 tablespoon of lite syrup contains fewer calories (95) than a bowl of Cheerios with milk (120 calories plus milk).

You're completely on your own for the first time, eating with friends in the cafeteria for breakfast, lunch, and dinner, often prolonging the meal by socializing. You're snacking in your room; because most dorms don't allow cooking, snack foods are easiest to store. Supermarkets may be inaccessible to you, forcing you to buy junk food at the campus convenience store. And everytime you turn around, someone's ordering pizza. By winter break, you've gained weight.

The good news is that your college roommates and other friends are going through it, too. And together, you can come up with some solutions. Organize an aerobics group or take an exercise class together. Play an intramural sport. Walk to class instead of taking the campus bus (or get off the bus a few stops early and walk the rest of the way). Or ride a bike! Make frequent use of the athletic center. Agree to help each other to limit high-calorie snacking to one or two nights a week or fewer. Use the Product Guide to learn which snacks are okay, and follow the guidelines in this book so you don't end up snacking five times a day instead of once or twice. And whatever you do, don't starve yourself to stay thinner by going on a crash diet. Even if your body is full grown, it still needs calories to perform efficiently. See your doctor to determine the appropriate weight goal for you, from among three options: weight slowdown, weight maintenance, and weight loss (only for full-grown teens or severely obese growing kids). Only your doctor will be able to tell you how much more growing you are likely to do, and what you should do about your weight now. Chapter 2 offers guidelines for this important medical visit.

CAUTION: Do not start this program without consulting your health care provider. Only your doctor can determine which weight-management goal and calorie level are right for you. If you try to do it yourself, without an initial doctor visit, you risk inhibiting your growth.

It's All in the Timing

If you're like most teens, you are active day to night, all week long, waking up early for school, going nonstop with classes, homework, activities, and socializing. On weekends, you may "crash," sleeping in and disrupting your eating schedule. Because you're so busy, you have many opportunities to snack throughout the day, opportunities you may not even think about, like eating chips as you study, grabbing an ice cream with a friend, drinking a soda at a sports event. And because you're becoming independent, making your own plans and spending your own money, it will be up to you to set limits. My menus (see pages 93–112) give you a framework for eating that includes three meals a day plus snacks. You can then decide for yourself if you want a dessert right after dinner or something to munch on later as you finish homework or watch a video. And when unexpected snacking opportunities arise— a class party, pizza with friends—you can remind yourself to give up one of your scheduled snacks in exchange. (Getting extra exercise that day also helps!) You really don't need to say no to the normal socializing that all teenagers enjoy. All it takes is some moderation, some give and take. In time, you'll find it becoming easier to set limits for yourself.

At Mom's House, At Dad's House

Taking control of your eating in your everyday environment is one thing, but what about the time you spend outside your usual routine? If your parents are divorced, you may confront some challenges when you spend a night, a weekend, or a vacation with the parent you see less often. Going out to eat may be a regular part of your visit, and it will be up to you to set some limits on what you order and how much you eat. If that parent lives far enough away from your other parent that you can't see your friends or visit your regular hang-outs, it may be easy to slip away from your everyday regimen. If you can, why not enlist the help of both parents? Talk about your new way of eating. Find out about exercise opportunities near each parent's home (local recreation classes, aerobics studios, even hiking trails). You can even make plans for some physical activity you can do together with each of them.

It's Up to You

Increasing independence is one of the perks of growing up. It is, as they say, a privilege and a responsibility. You have the privilege of making more of your own decisions. And you have a responsibility to make the best decisions you can. For this reason, I encourage adolescents to be in charge of their own weight management. You're not a kid anymore, and you don't need your mom and dad to play "food police" while you get annoyed and try to undermine them. It's too easy for you to get those extra calories when you're out and about. And it's wrong for your parents to battle with you over what you ate when, and how much. Make this *your* project. After all, you are the one who will benefit.

It's certainly fine to ask for support from your parents as you embark on this lifestyle change, however. Here are some ways your parents can help you:

- Have your parents make an appointment with your doctor, who can perform a physical examination to see where things stand right now and help you select a weight-management goal and a calorie level.
- Ask whichever parent does the grocery shopping and meal preparation to look over the menus and Product Guide with you. Make a list of the items you want to keep around the house for your breakfasts, lunches, and snacks. (If you drive, perhaps your parent would allow you to go out and purchase the items yourself.)
- Talk about ways to get exercise, such as taking a class, working out with an exercise video, riding a bicycle, and so on. Discuss which options appeal to you, and how often they will be available. You will want to exercise three or

more times a week for at least thirty minutes per session, so be sure to choose something you'll be able to do regularly.

Your parents want to be an emotional support for you. But don't ask them to be your keepers. If you aren't ready to make a change, there's nothing your parents can do to make you watch your weight. Temptations are everywhere. That's why you'll have to take charge. This is your chance to be independent, using this book as your guide. Don't rely on your parents to tell you no. Those days are over. Now it's up to you.

INDEX